Illustrated Signs in Clinical Paediatrics

For information on Churchill Livingstone titles, or to place an order, call

UK: Freephone 0500 566 242
Europe: + 44 131 535 1021
USA/Canada: + 1 201 319 9800
Australia/New Zealand: + 61 3 9699 5400

Illustrated Signs in Clinical Paediatrics

A Minford MB ChB, DCH, FRCP, FRCPCH
Consultant Paediatrician,
St Luke's Hospital, Bradford, UK

R Arumugam DCH MD MRCP(UK)
Fellow, Division of Gastroenterology and Nutrition,
Texas Children's Hospital and Baylor College of Medicine, Houston, Texas, USA

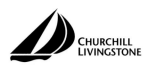

CHURCHILL
LIVINGSTONE

NEW YORK EDINBURGH LONDON MADRID MELBOURNE
SAN FRANCISCO AND TOKYO 1998

CHURCHILL LIVINGSTONE
Medical Division of Pearson Professional Limited

Distributed in the United States of America by Churchill
Livingstone Inc., 650 Avenue of the Americas, New York,
N.Y. 10011, and by associated companies, branches and
representatives throughout the world.

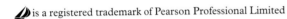
First published 1998

ISBN 0 443 05529 7

British Library Cataloguing in Publication Data
A catalogue record for this book is available from the
British Library.

Library of Congress Cataloging in Publication Data
A catalog record for this book is available from the Library
of Congress.

Medical knowledge is constantly changing. As new
information becomes available, changes in treatment,
procedures, equipment and the use of drugs become
necessary. The authors and the publishers have, as far as it
is possible, taken care to ensure that the information given
in this text is accurate and up to date. However, readers are
strongly advised to confirm that the information, especially
with regard to drug usage, complies with current legislation
and standards of practice.

The
publisher's
policy is to use
**paper manufactured
from sustainable forests**

Produced by Longman Asia Limited, Hong Kong.
GCC/01

Preface

The majority of commonly occurring as well as some rare paediatric conditions and physical signs are included in this comprehensive collection of clinical illustrations. A brief description is provided for each illustration, giving the most salient points relating to the particular condition or signs as well as identifying associated symptoms.

The aim of the book is to provide an essential visual aid which can be used in conjunction with more traditional paediatric texts. We hope that undergraduates as well as those reading for higher paediatric examinations will find the book a useful and invaluable source of illustrative reference for revision and will be encouraged to develop their practical recognition skills.

A M   Bradford   1998
R A   Texas   1998

Acknowledgements

We are grateful to Mrs Carol Fleming and her staff of the Medical Illustration Department of St. Luke's Hospital for providing many of the clinical photographs and to Valerie Williams and Wendy Misaljevich for secretarial assistance.

We would also like to thank the following colleagues who generously provided photographs: Dr Malcolm Arthurton, Dr Geoff Lealman, Dr David Haigh, Dr Steve Green, Dr Chris Day, Dr Sue Chatfield, Dr Peter Corry, Dr D Subesinghe, Dr Andrew Wright, Dr Derek Barker, Dr Jim Littlewood, Dr Keith Brown, Professor Bob Mueller, Mr Mike Timmons, Mr Chris Raine, Mr John Bradbury, Mr Mark Stringer, Dr Philip Helliwell, Dr Alan Watson and Dr David Curnock.

Contents

1 Head and neck

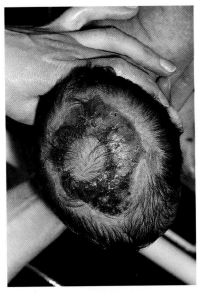

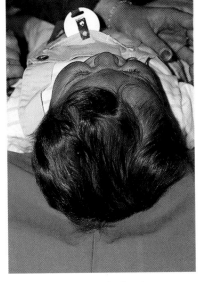

Fig. 1 Aplasia cutis congenita   **Fig. 2 Plagiocephaly**

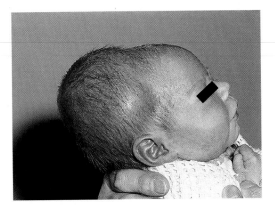

Fig. 3 Cephalhaematoma

Fig. 1 Aplasia cutis congenita consists of localised areas of congenitally absent skin which are most frequently found on the scalp. An ulcerated area is present at birth and this heals leaving a scar. Other congenital abnormalities may be present, e.g. limb reductions, myelomeningocele and malformation syndromes.

Fig. 2 The head is asymmetrical with flattening of the right occipital region. Plagiocephaly is usually postural in origin and is associated with a strong preference to look to one side (the right side in this case). Facial asymmetry is often associated with this condition, and occasionally there may be thoracic asymmetry. The condition resolves gradually with age, except in handicapped children in whom asymmetry may be permanent.

Fig. 3 There is a large boggy swelling over the parietal bone due to subperiosteal haemorrhage. Cephalhaematoma, which is always limited to a single cranial bone, appears a few hours after birth and resolves spontaneously, sometimes with calcification, over a few months. Occasionally, there is an underlying fracture, but hyperbilirubinaemia is the commonest neonatal complication.

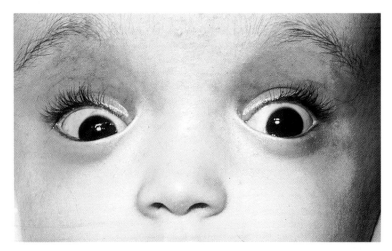

Fig. 4 Sunsetting sign

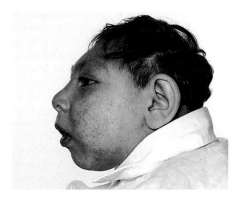

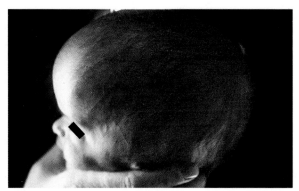

Fig. 5 Microcephaly   **Fig. 6 Hydranencephaly**

Fig. 4 The sclera are visible between the iris and the upper eyelid. The sunsetting sign, which is seen most often in hydrocephalus, is due to loss of upward conjugate gaze caused by raised intracranial pressure.

Fig. 5 Microcephaly is usually defined as a head circumference which is more than three standard deviations below the mean for age and sex. In this gross example, the forehead is slanted and the ears appear disproportionately large. Gross microcephaly is often autosomal recessive in its inheritance and is associated with severe mental retardation. It may also be a feature of syndromes (e.g. Cri-du-chat) or secondary to intrauterine infection or hypoxic-ischaemic encephalopathy.

Fig. 6 In hydranencephaly, the cerebral hemispheres are absent but the midbrain and brain stem are intact. At birth the head circumference is normal or increased, but postnatal growth is excessive. Absence of the hemispheres can be demonstrated by transillumination, as shown above. This is a sporadic condition and the aetiology is unknown.

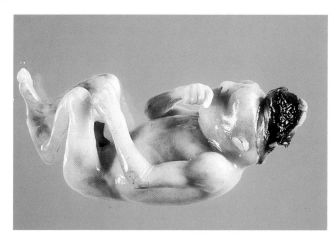

Fig. 7 Anencephaly

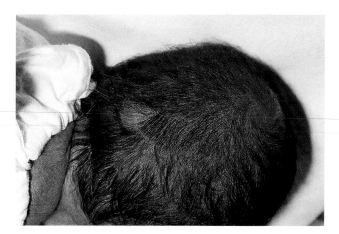

Fig. 8 Encephalocele

Fig. 7 Anencephaly is characterised by a large defect of the skull and scalp with a very rudimentary brain. Most affected infants die within a few days of birth. Women who have had anencephalic infants should have subsequent pregnancies closely monitored, with determination of alpha fetoprotein levels and ultrasound examination. Fortunately, neural tube defects have become less common in recent years due to folic acid supplementation.

Fig. 8 An encephalocele is a midline, usually occipital, defect through which meninges and brain have herniated. Frontal and nasopharyngeal encephaloceles also occur but are less common. Neurological problems such as mental retardation, visual impairment and seizures are common, and hydrocephalus may occur.

Fig. 9 Holoprosencephaly

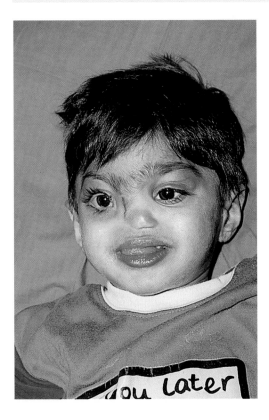

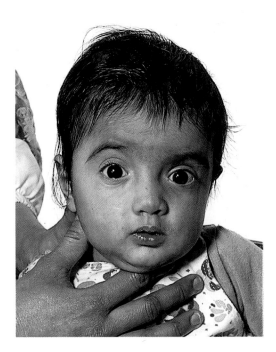

Fig. 10 Craniosynostosis

Fig. 9 Holoprosencephaly refers to failure of the forebrain (prosencephalon) to divide into two cerebral hemispheres. There may be accompanying midline facial abnormalities. The child shown above has an abnormally flat nasal bridge and a single nostril.

Fig. 10 This girl with craniosynostosis has unilateral flattening of the forehead (frontal plagiocephaly) and depression of the orbit due to premature fusion of the right coronal suture. Surgical treatment usually gives a good result in such cases.

Fig. 11 Cyanosis

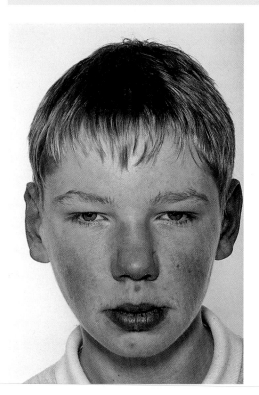

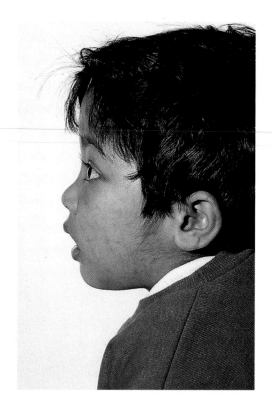

Fig. 12 Thalassaemia

Fig. 11 This boy has central cyanosis due to right to left shunting as a result of congenital cyanotic heart disease. Peripheral cyanosis is often present in young children when cold. This must be differentiated from central cyanosis in which blueness is observed in the tongue and mucous membranes.

Fig. 12 Facial features due to bone marrow expansion, including frontal bossing and maxillary enlargement with protruding upper frontal teeth, should not be seen in the adequately treated child with thalassaemia major. This boy with thalassaemia intermedia had a prominent maxilla before a programme of regular blood transfusions was started due to a fall-off in growth.

Fig. 13 Bernard Soulier syndrome

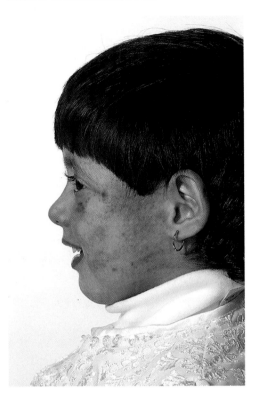

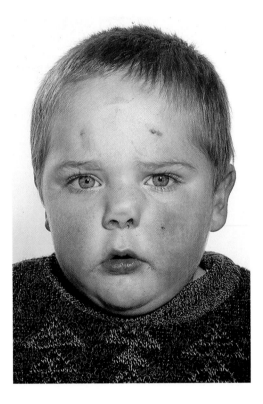

Fig. 14 Atonic seizures

Fig. 13 Bernard Soulier syndrome is a disorder of platelet function which can cause extensive bruising, and sometimes these children are referred as cases of non-accidental injury (NAI). This girl sustained superficial bruising after vigorous playing with her friends. Such cases illustrate the importance of always performing coagulation tests, including bleeding time, in all suspected cases of NAI.

Fig. 14 This boy shows evidence of repeated facial injury from atonic seizures. He refused to wear his protective helmet for several years. He also suffered from myoclonic jerks and absence attacks, and his epilepsy was refractory to treatment with anticonvulsant drugs.

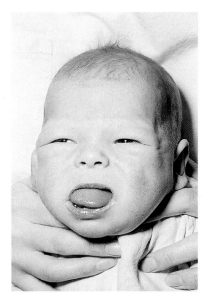

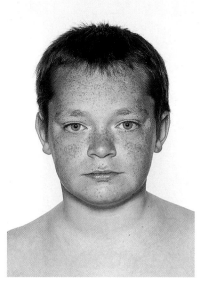

Fig. 15 Congenital hypothyroidism

Fig. 16 Acquired hypothyroidism

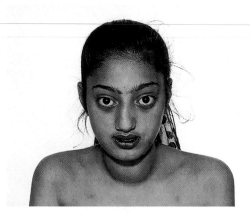

Fig. 17 Thyrotoxicosis

Fig. 15 This baby has macroglossia and coarse facial features. With the advent of neonatal screening, this appearance should rarely, if ever, be seen today. The clinical features of congenital hypothyroidism include feeding difficulties, hoarse cry, sluggishness, respiratory difficulties, thickened cold skin, constipation, slow heart rate, umbilical hernia and prolonged neonatal jaundice.

Fig. 16 This boy presented with marked slowing of growth velocity and tiredness. The signs of classical hypothyroidism and myxoedema are rare in children and, other than short stature, the only clinical signs in this boy were dry skin and slight enlargement of the thyroid gland. Autoimmune thyroiditis is almost always the cause of acquired hypothyroidism.

Fig. 17 This girl with hyperthyroidism has a goitre, exophthalmos and an anxious expression. Children with hyperthyroidism may present with school problems (short attention span), tall stature, weight loss with increased appetite and the effects of a hyperactive sympathetic nervous system. Exophthalmos tends to be milder than in adults and is preceded by lid lag on looking downwards and upper eyelid retraction.

Fig. 18 Dystrophia myotonica

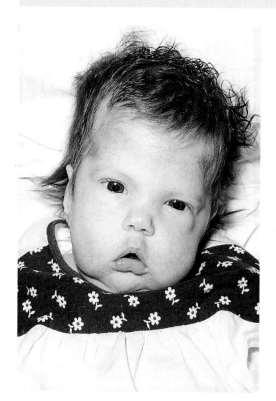

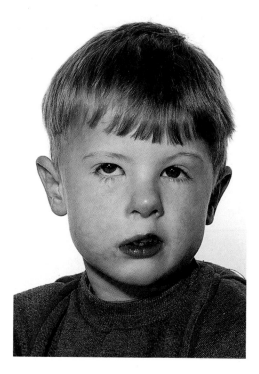

Fig. 19 Möbius syndrome

Fig. 18 This girl, whose mother also had dystrophia myotonica, suffered from the more severe neo-natal form of the condition. She shows an expressionless myopathic facies with a characteristic open tent-shaped mouth. Typically, she had severe generalised hypotonia and weakness from birth, and required prolonged ventilator support. Neonatal myotonic dystrophy has a significant early mortality and learning difficulties are common in survivors.

Fig. 19 The features of Möbius syndrome are congenital facial paresis and sixth nerve weakness. Facial weakness is usually bilateral but often incomplete and asymmetrical. The upper part of the face may be relatively unaffected. Sixth cranial nerve weakness may be unilateral or bilateral. The syndrome is thought to be due to agenesis of cranial nerve nuclei.

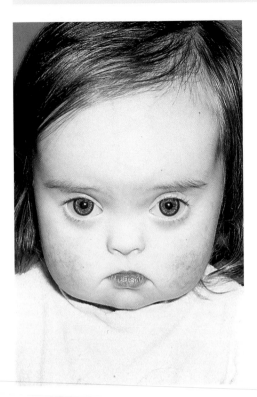

Fig. 20 Trisomy 21

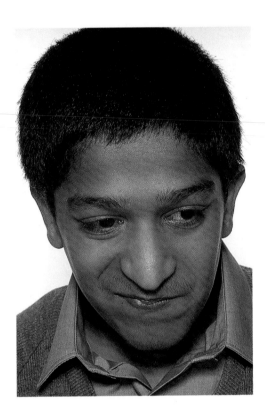

Fig. 21 Fragile X syndrome

Fig. 20 This girl with Trisomy 21 shows several characteristic facial features - hypertelorism, Brushfield spots, upward-slanting palpebral fissures, depressed nasal bridge, full cheeks and small mouth.

Fig. 21 This boy with learning difficulties has a long face with coarse features and prognathism. Other phenotypic features of fragile X syndrome include large everted ears and macro-orchidism. This syndrome is variable in its clinical features and 10% of affected males have normal facial features. It is the commonest single cause of inherited mental retardation.

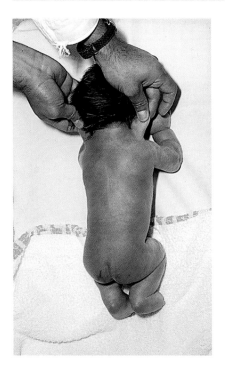

Fig. 22a Turner syndrome

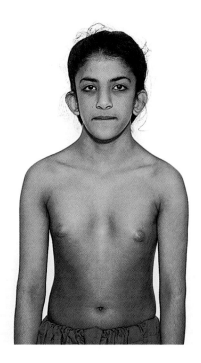

Fig. 22b Turner syndrome

Fig. 22a–b (**a**) This baby has loose skin folds at the side of her neck. This sign and oedema of the hands and feet are the most obvious features of Turner syndrome in the neonatal period. However, there may be no obvious clinical features at this time, the patient presenting later with short stature. (**b**) Dysmorphic features may be minimal in girls with Turner syndrome. This girl has protruding ears, slight pectus excavatum and widely spaced nipples, but she does not have classical webbing of the neck or cubitus valgus. She presented with short stature. Chromosome analysis should always be part of the investigation of girls who are small for their mid-parent height, even though they have none of the typical features of Turner syndrome.

Fig. 23 Noonan syndrome

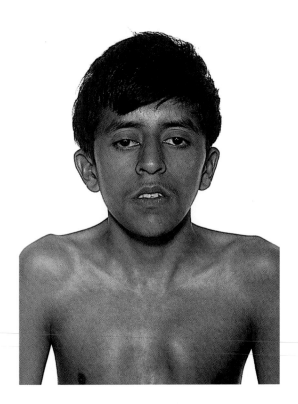

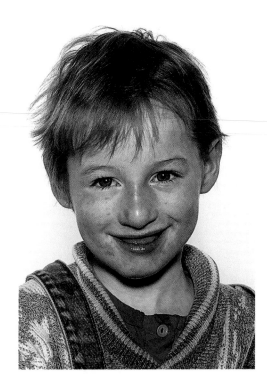

Fig. 24 Angelman syndrome

Fig. 23 This boy with short stature, learning difficulties and pulmonary stenosis shows several of the features of Noonan syndrome – low set ears, ptosis of the eyelids, short neck and pectus excavatum. Other features of this syndrome, which are not evident in this patient, include epicanthic folds, down-slanting palpable fissures, hypertelorism, webbed neck and cryptorchidism.

Fig. 24 The typical facial phenotype of Angelman syndrome is shown – wide smiling mouth, thin upper lip, pointed prominent chin and fair hair. Other features of this syndrome are severe mental handicap, epilepsy, a happy disposition and ataxic gait with the arms held flexed at the elbow. This condition was formerly known as the 'happy puppet syndrome'.

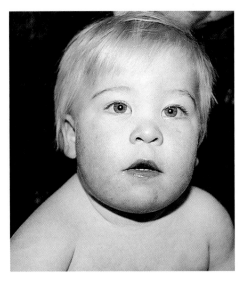

Fig. 25 Prader–Willi syndrome

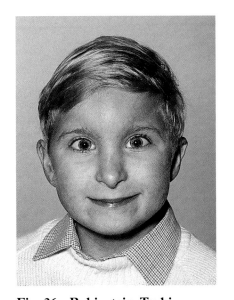

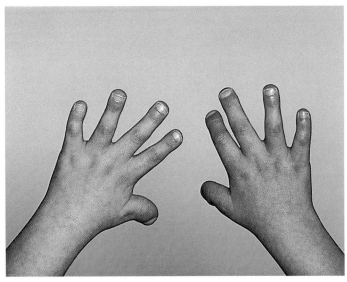

Fig. 26a Rubinstein–Taybi syndrome

Fig. 26b Rubenstein–Taybi syndrome

Fig. 25 This boy has almond-shaped palpebral fissures, fair hair, a narrow bifrontal diameter and obesity, which are all characteristic of Prader–Willi syndrome. These children also have marked hypotonia in early infancy, mental retardation, short stature, small hands and feet, and small genitalia. The syndrome is associated with a deletion of chromosome 15 at the q 11–13 region.

Fig. 26a–b (**a**) This boy shows several of the facial features of Rubinstein–Taybi syndrome – beaked nose with nasal septum extending below the alae nasi, low set ears and hypoplastic mandible. He also has short stature and severe learning difficulties, which are characteristic of the syndrome. (**b**) Short broad thumbs with radial angulation occur in virtually all patients with this syndrome. All this patient's fingers are short, and the toes are similarly affected.

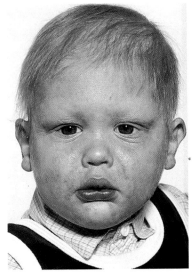

Fig. 27a Hypohidrotic ectodermal dysplasia

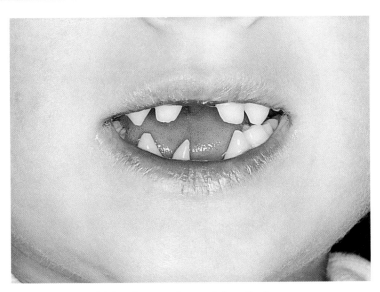

Fig. 27b Hypohidrotic ectodermal dysplasia

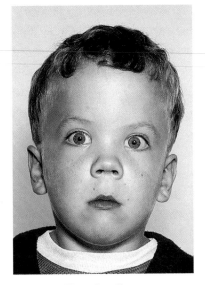

Fig. 28a Basal cell naevus syndrome

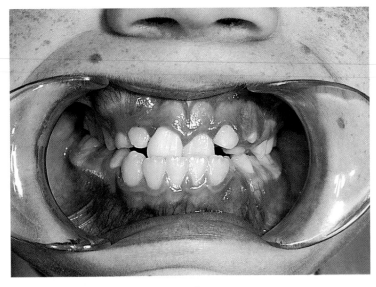

Fig. 28b Basal cell naevus syndrome

Fig. 27a–b (a) This boy has several of the facial features of hypohidrotic ectodermal dysplasia – sparse fine hair, frontal bossing, sparse eyebrows, a sunken nasal bridge, thin wrinkled skin around his eyes and a thick protruding lower lip. Hypoplasia of the sweat glands may lead to hyperthermia, and absence or hypoplasia of mucous glands may be responsible for an increased susceptibility to respiratory infection. (b) Hypodontia with abnormal, often peg-shaped or conical teeth or adontia are characteristic of this condition. Inheritance is X-linked, but about 10% of heterozygous females show features of the syndrome. This patient is the sister of the boy shown in (a). Apart from abnormal teeth and thin hair, she has no other features.

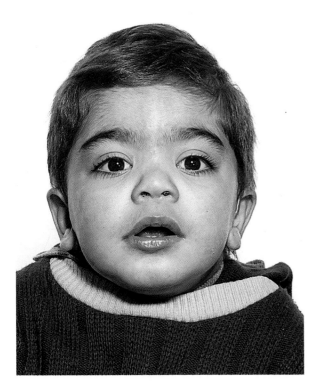

Fig. 29 Sanfilippo syndrome

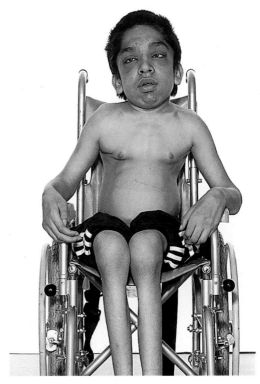

Fig. 30 Hurler–Sheie syndrome

Fig. 28a–b (opposite) (**a**) This boy shows the characteristic facial appearance of basal cell naevus syndrome (Gorlin syndrome) – large head size due to frontal and biparietal bulging, broadened nasal root, mild hypertelorism and increased mandibular length. The other major manifestations of this syndrome are naevoid basal cell carcinomata developing after puberty, odontogenic keratocysts of the jaw and other tumours, especially of the central nervous system. (**b**) At the age of 11 years, this patient was found to have multiple odontogenic keratocysts of the mandible and maxilla. These develop in over 80% of patients. A cyst is visible above the gum on the right side. These cysts may loosen the teeth, extend to soft tissues and invade sinuses.

Fig. 29 Sanfilippo syndrome (mucopolysaccharidosis type III) is the commonest mucopolysacchari-dosis disorder and is associated with excessive urinary excretion of heparan sulphate. This child has a slightly coarse facial appearance with a depressed nasal bridge and short neck, but the coarse facial features and skeletal abnormalities are milder than those seen in Hurler's syndrome. These children have severe learning difficulties, and rapid neurological deterioration is the usual course. Most patients die in their mid-teens.

Fig. 30 Hurler–Scheie syndrome is a mucopolysaccharide disorder due to L-iduronidase deficiency. Dermatan sulphate is stored in the liver, spleen and other tissues, and excreted in the urine. The features shown by this patient include coarseness of facial features, corneal clouding, short stature and joint contractures. Hepatosplenomegaly and heart valve lesions also occur, but unlike Hurler's syndrome mental retardation is not a feature and long-term survival can occur.

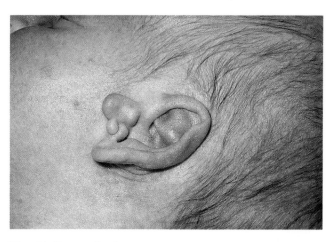

Fig. 31 Preauricular tags

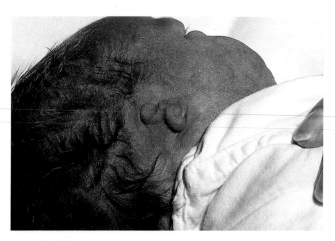

Fig. 32 Microtia

Fig. 31 Several broad-based skin tags are present in front of the ear. Skin tags with a narrow pedicle can be ligated, but broad-based tags require surgical excision. Malformations of the external ear may sometimes be associated with renal or other congenital abnormalities.

Fig. 32 There is malformation of the external ear in this child with the Treacher–Collins syndrome (mandibulofacial dysostosis). Rudimentary auricles result from developmental abnormalities of the first and second branchial arches. In addition to mandibulofacial dysostosis, other associations include middle ear abnormalities, other craniofacial abnormalities and renal anomalies.

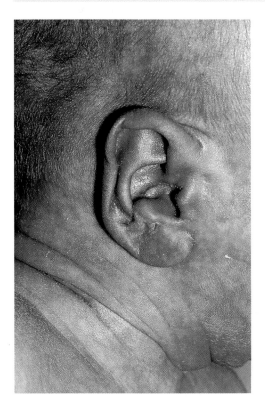

Fig. 33 Beckwith–Wiedemann syndrome

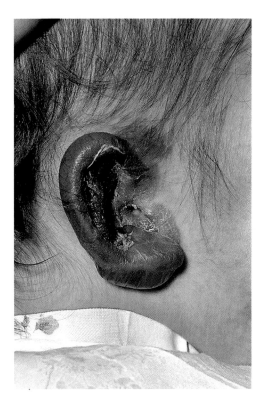

Fig. 34 Cellulitis of the auricle

Fig. 33 Linear creases are present in the earlobe of this baby who had exomphalos at birth. The other features of Beckwith–Wiedemann syndrome are high birth weight, macroglossia, visceromegaly, microcephaly and hypoglycaemia (often severe) associated with hyperinsulinism. The condition is usually sporadic, although familial cases have occurred.

Fig. 34 The auricle and adjacent skin of this immunosuppressed child are red, hot, swollen and painful. The external auditory canal is also involved. Haemolytic streptococci, and sometimes *Staphylococcus aureus*, are the usual pathogens.

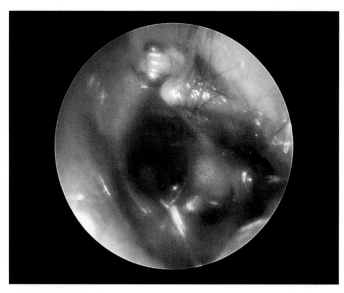

Fig. 35 Secretory otitis media (glue ear)

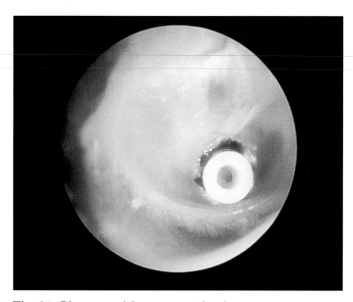

Fig. 36 Glue ear with grommet in situ

Fig. 35 Fluid is seen behind the left tympanic membrane. The fluid may appear as amber or dark blue, and air bubbles or an air–fluid level may also be present. Glue ear is a common condition which causes conductive hearing loss. It is usually painless and should be excluded when parents or teachers express concern about a child's hearing.

Fig. 36 A small tube (grommet) has been inserted into the tympanic membrane of this child with glue ear to improve ventilation of the middle ear and prevent reaccumulation of fluid. This procedure is usually followed by marked improvement in hearing.

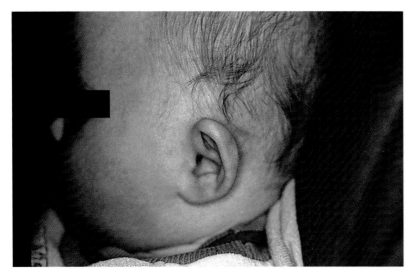

Fig. 37 Mastoiditis

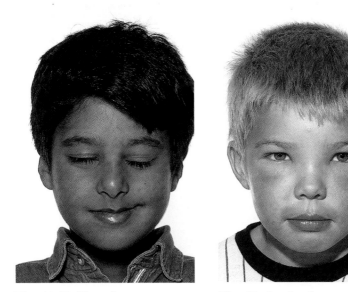

Fig. 38 Bell's palsy   **Fig. 39 Angioedema**

Fig. 37 There is redness and swelling over the left mastoid process. Mastoiditis usually results from acute otitis media and causes the ear to be displaced forwards and downwards.

Fig. 38 This boy developed right-sided facial weakness 2 weeks after a viral illness. When asked to smile and close his eyes, the right side of his face is immobile and eye closure is incomplete. His prognosis is excellent and, other than corneal protection with eye drops, no treatment is indicated.

Fig. 39 Swelling of the eyelids and lips (angioedema) are seen in this boy with urticaria. Causes include infection, drugs, food allergy and insect bites, although often the responsible agent is unknown. Periorbital oedema is also a presenting feature of glomerulonephritis and nephrotic syndrome. Therefore, urine testing is essential before attributing the cause to allergy.

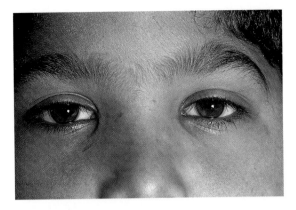

Fig. 40 Epicanthic folds

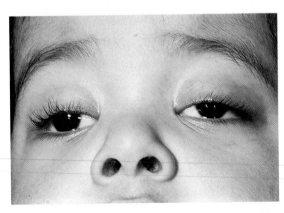

Fig. 41a Myasthenia gravis

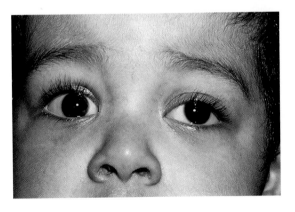

Fig. 41b Myasthenia gravis

Fig. 40 Folds of skin covering the inner canthus of each eye are present. These are often seen in very young children but disappear with age. They can give the impression of a squint. Although not rare in normal older children, they are common in a large number of syndromes, e.g. trisomy 21.

Fig. 41a–b Ocular muscles are very frequently involved in children with myasthenia gravis. (**a**) This boy presented with ptosis, which was characteristically worse towards the end of the day. The diagnosis was confirmed by demonstrating reversal of his eye signs after intravenous injection of edrophonium. (**b**) This is the same patient after 2 weeks of treatment with pyridostigmine. In myasthenia gravis, antibodies to acetylcholine receptors cause neuromuscular block which can be reversed by anticholinesterases.

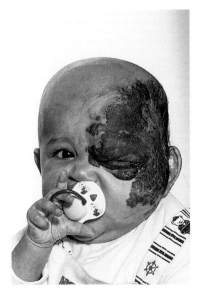

Fig. 42 Periorbital haemangioma

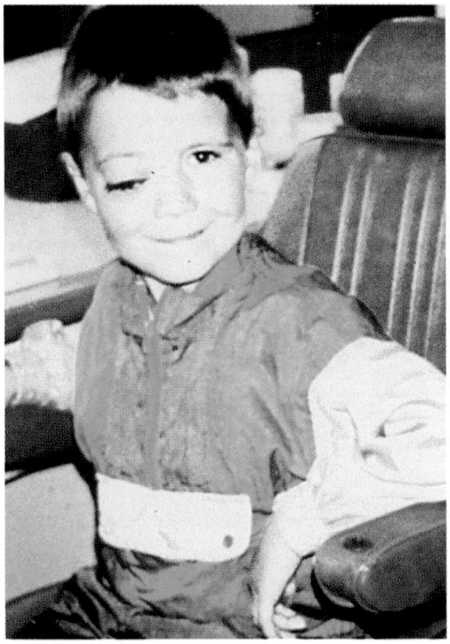

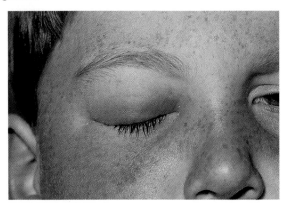

Fig. 43 Proptosis

Fig. 44 Periorbital cellulitis

Fig. 42 Not all haemangiomas are benign in their effects. A periorbital haemangioma may obstruct vision, leading to amblyopia, and should be treated. Steroids may hasten involution. Large haemangiomas may also compress airways, cause high output cardiac failure and cause consumption coagulopathy (Kasabach–Merritt syndrome).

Fig. 43 This child's right eye is displaced forwards and downwards by an orbital rhabdomyosarcoma. This child's proptosis is quite obvious, but in the early stages this clinical sign is best elicited by noting asymmetry when viewing from above. Unilateral proptosis is usually due to a neoplasm, e.g. rhabdomyosarcoma or metastases from a neuroblastoma.

Fig. 44 Swelling and erythema of the eyelids and adjacent soft tissues of the face occurred in this boy as a result of spread from sinus infection. Periorbital cellulitis is potentially serious and may lead to cavernous sinus thrombosis, orbital cellulitis with orbital pain, impaired vision and loss of ocular movement. *Haemophilus influenzae* is the commonest responsible organism.

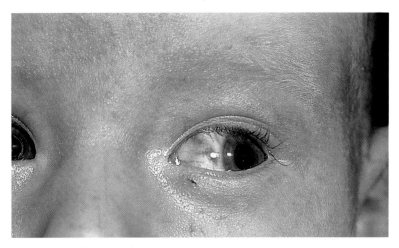

Fig. 45 Conjunctival haemorrhage

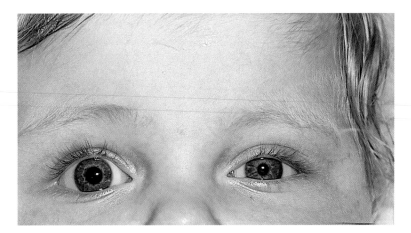

Fig. 46 Horner syndrome

Fig. 45 Conjunctival haemorrhage and a few petechiae around the eye are present in this child with pertussis. These occur as a result of raised intrathoracic pressure during coughing paroxysms. The same mechanism may also produce upper body petechiae, epistaxis, retinal haemorrhage and haemorrhage in the central nervous system.

Fig. 46 The left eye shows the characteristic features of Horner syndrome – miosis, ptosis and enophthalmos. Ipsilateral anhidrosis of the face is the other feature. The syndrome is due to paresis of the ocular sympathetic nerve supply. Causes include birth trauma, cardiac surgery and mediastinal or cervical tumours, e.g. neuroblastoma. Sometimes no cause is identified.

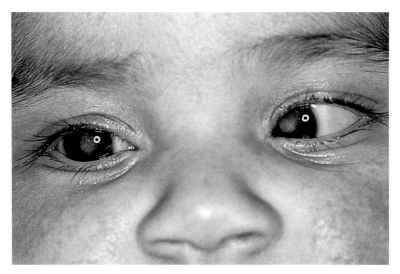

Fig. 47 Leucocoria

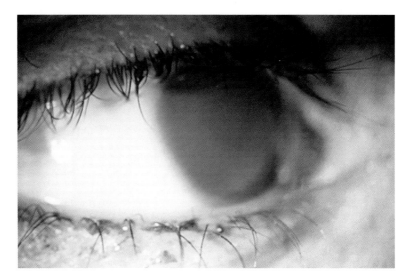

Fig. 48 Corneal opacity

Fig. 47 This blind girl has strabismus and bilateral white pupils as a result of organising vitreous haemorrhage. Assessment of the red light reflex is an essential part of eye examination. Its absence and the presence of a white pupil indicate serious intraocular pathology such as retinoblastoma, cataract or retinal detachment.

Fig. 48 Cloudiness of the cornea is present. Corneal opacity is seen in congenital glaucoma and in some of the mucopolysaccharidoses or may be the result of injury or inflammation.

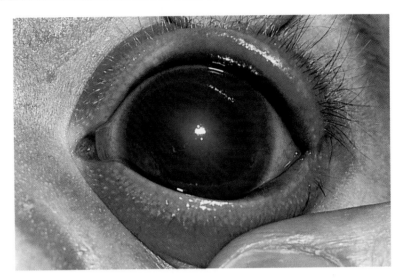

Fig. 49 Glaucoma

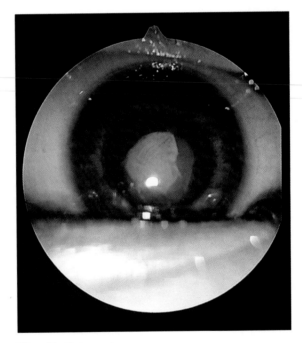

Fig. 50 Cataract

Fig. 49 The cornea is enlarged and hazy in this patient with congenital glaucoma. Infants usually present with photophobia or the parents may notice that the eye appears large. The corneal diameter usually exceeds 12 mm. Urgent referral to an ophthalmologist is indicated.

Fig. 50 A dense lens opacity is present in this child with congenital cataract. Cataract may be due to intrauterine infection, metabolic disease (e.g. galactosaemia), chromosomal defects (e.g. trisomy 21), prematurity, corticosteroids and trauma, and occurs in a large number of syndromes.

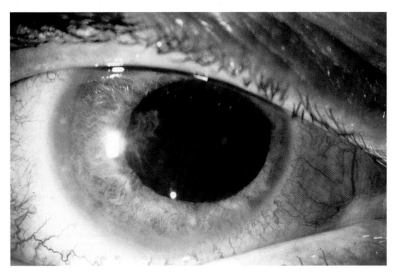

Fig. 51 Lens dislocation

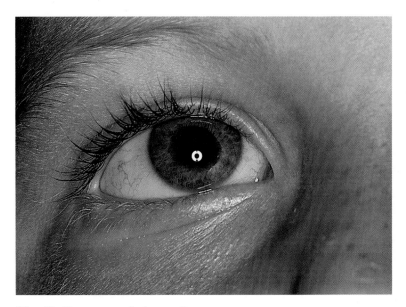

Fig. 52 Osteogenesis imperfecta

Fig. 51 Lateral displacement of the lens secondary to trauma is seen. Dislocation can also occur secondary to intraocular disease, such as glaucoma, or as an isolated abnormality. In Marfan syndrome the lens is usually displaced superiorly and temporally, while in homocystinuria it is usually displaced inferiorally and nasally.

Fig. 52 Blueness of the sclera is a characteristic feature of autosomal dominant type I osteogenesis imperfecta, but in the more severe recessively inherited type III, the sclera are usually white. It is important to remember that normal neonates may have a slightly blue hue to their sclera.

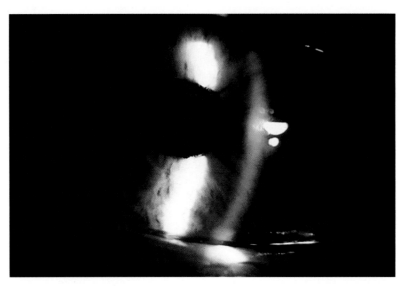

Fig. 53 Lisch nodules

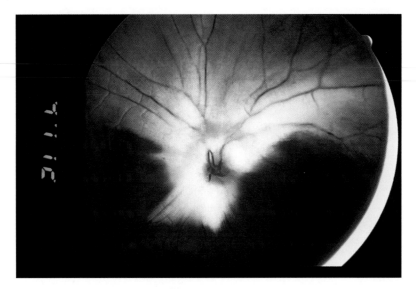

Fig. 54 Myelinated nerve fibres

Fig. 53 Slit lamp examination is usually necessary to see Lisch nodules clearly. They are small, slightly elevated pigmented lesions of the iris in patients with neurofibromatosis. They are asymptomatic, but their presence is helpful when the diagnosis of neurofibromatosis is in doubt.

Fig. 54 There is an extensive white area running outwards from the optic disc caused by myelination of the retinal nerve fibres. Normally, myelination ends at the optic disc. The perimeter of the myelinated area often has a feathery appearance. The macula is usually unaffected in this condition, so that vision is often quite good although there may be a visual field defect. If the abnormality is extensive, the child may have myopia or strabismus.

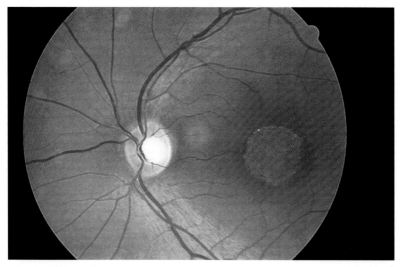

Fig. 55 Cone dystrophy

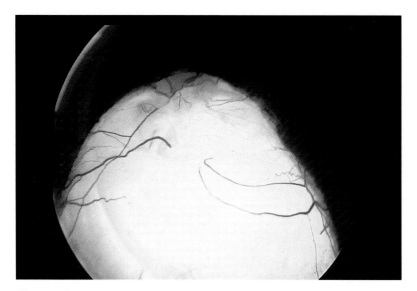

Fig. 56 Coloboma of the fundus

Fig. 55 A typical 'bull's eye' appearance is seen at the macula in this case of cone dystrophy. This condition may be sporadic or dominantly inherited and is characterised by photophobia with progressive loss of central vision and colour vision. On visual field testing, a small central scotoma is often detected but peripheral visual fields remain intact.

Fig. 56 In coloboma of the fundus, an extensive well-demarcated white area is present which engulfs the optic disc and exposes underlying sclera. Visual acuity is likely to be impaired with such a large defect. Colobomata of the fundus may occur as isolated defects or may occur with other ocular abnormalities such as microphthalmia. They may also occur in chromosome abnormalities (e.g. trisomy 13 and 18) and in a number of syndromes (e.g. Aicardi, Rubinstein–Taybi).

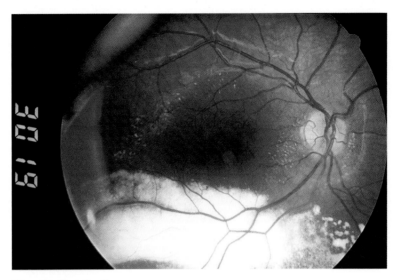

Fig. 57 Coat's disease

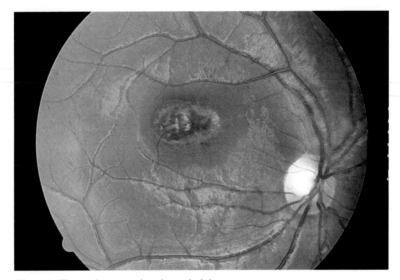

Fig. 58 Toxoplasma chorioretinitis

Fig. 57 In Coat's disease, there is extensive exudate into the retina resulting from leakage of plasma from telangiectatic retinal vessels. This non-familial condition predominantly affects boys who are otherwise well. It is usually unilateral and presents with blurred vision, squint or leucocoria. Complications include retinal detachment and glaucoma.

Fig. 58 An area of chorioretinitis is present, consisting of scarring surrounded by pigmentation. Most cases of ocular toxoplasmosis are believed to be the result of congenital infection. The majority of children with congenital toxoplasma infection will develop chorioretinitis, although this may be delayed until later childhood or adolescence.

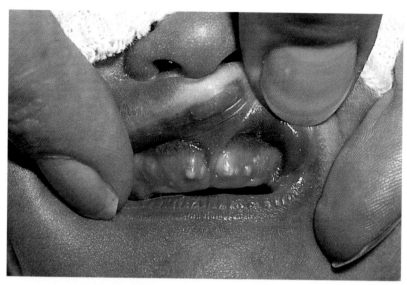

Fig. 59 Epithelial pearls

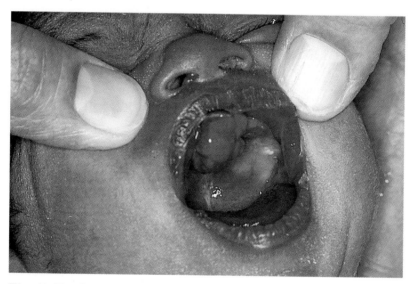

Fig. 60 Epulis

Fig. 59 These common small inclusion cysts can be seen on the alveolar margins of the neonate. Epstein's pearls are clusters of these lesions occurring at the junction of the hard and soft palate in the midline. These lesions soon fade and attempts should not be made to remove them.

Fig. 60 In neonates, epulis, a tumour-like growth of the gums, is most often found in the maxillary incisor region and appears as a mass on the alveolar margin. Treatment is by surgical excision. These lesions do not metastasise.

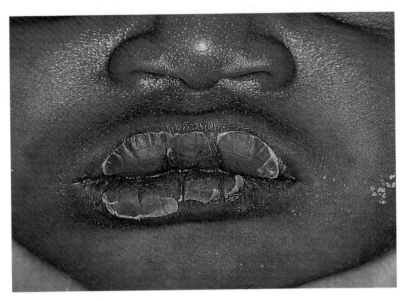

Fig. 61 Sucking pads

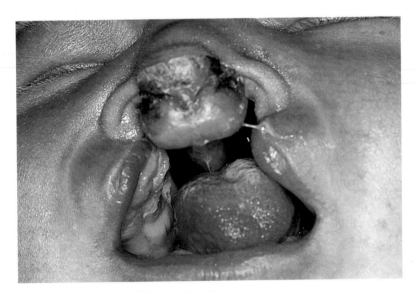

Fig. 62 Bilateral cleft lip and palate

Fig. 61 Sucking pads appear on the lips a few days after birth and have been seen in babies who have never sucked. After the pads are shed, new ones may appear for a few weeks.

Fig. 62 There are bilateral clefts involving the alveolar ridge with protrusion of the intermaxillary process. The clefts extend backwards, involving the hard and soft palate and exposing the nasal cavity. In the newborn period, the main problems are feeding, the possibility of other congenital abnormalities and parental reassurance.

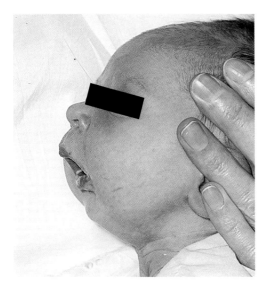

Fig. 63a Pierre Robin syndrome

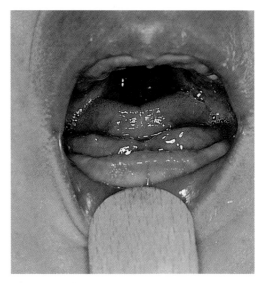

Fig. 63b Pierre Robin syndrome

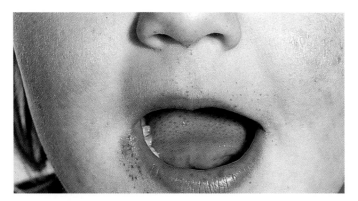

Fig. 64 Peutz–Jeghers syndrome

Fig. 63a–b (**a**) This infant has obvious micrognathia. The tongue is displaced backwards obstruct-ing the pharynx. Serious upper airway obstruction can occur, especially in the supine position, and the infant should be nursed in the prone position. This threat lessens after a few months as the mandible grows. The eventual profile after a period of about 5 years is often virtually normal. (**b**) Micrognathia is usually accompanied by a cleft palate, but this is not invariable and sometimes the palate may be high-arched without a cleft.

Fig. 64 Pigmented macules are seen around the mouth of this child with Peutz–Jeghers syndrome, an autosomal dominant condition. Similar lesions often occur on the buccal mucosa, and occasion-ally on the palm, soles and fingers. Gastrointestinal polyps may cause abdominal pain, intussuscep-tion and bleeding. Malignant change in the polyps is rare.

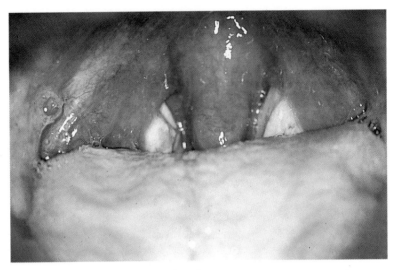

Fig. 65 Infectious mononucleosis

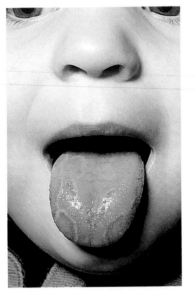

Fig. 66 Geographic tongue

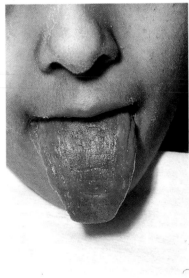

Fig. 67 Glossitis

Fig. 65 In cases of infectious mononucleosis, the tonsils are enlarged and coated with a creamy white exudate. The pillars of the tonsils and uvula are red and hyperaemic. Petechiae at the junction of the hard and soft palate is also a common finding. A membranous exudate may also occur in streptococcal infection and diphtheria.

Fig. 66 Smooth, red plaques with pale, slightly elevated margins are seen on the dorsum of this geographic tongue. The plaques which occur because of desquamation of the papillae are migratory and form map-like patterns. Irritation may occur with hot foods and drinks. No treatment is necessary.

Fig. 67 This patient with glossitis has a smooth, red, painful tongue with loss of papillae as a result of dietary deficiency of the vitamin B complex.

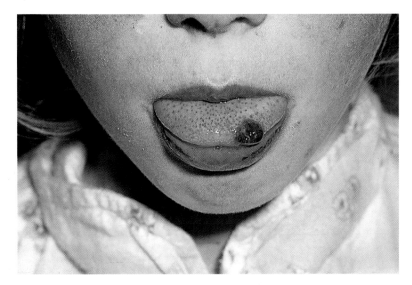

Fig. 68 Idiopathic thrombocytopenic purpura

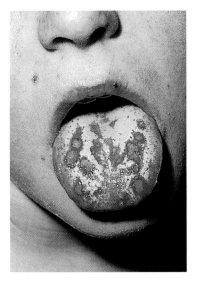

Fig. 69 Erythema multiforme

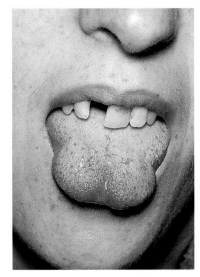

Fig. 70 Dystrophia myotonica

Fig. 68 In this girl a small haematoma has developed on the tongue. Most children with idiopathic thrombocytopenic purpura have superficial bruising and petechiae. Bleeding from mucous membranes is less common and serious internal bleeding, e.g. intracranial haemorrhage, is rare.

Fig. 69 Mucosal involvement affecting the tongue is seen in this child who had typical skin lesions of erythema multiforme. Infections, especially herpes simplex and mycoplasma, are the commonest causes in children. When skin lesions are extensive and severe, and at least two mucous membranes are involved, the condition is known as the Stevens–Johnson syndrome.

Fig. 70 In addition to demonstrating myotonica when shaking a patient's hand and when tapping the thenar eminence, this sign may also be demonstrated by tapping the patient's tongue, which can be seen to contract.

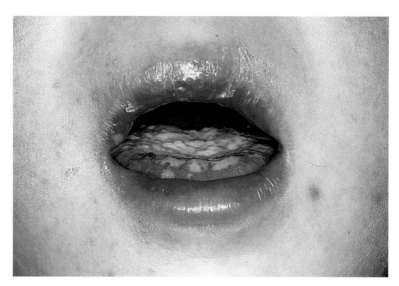

Fig. 71 Herpetic stomatitis

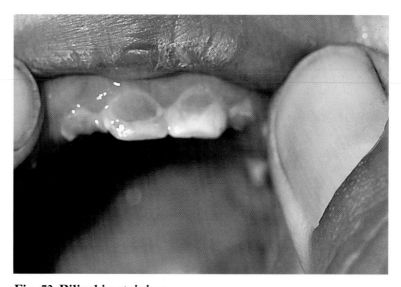

Fig. 72 Bilirubin staining

Fig. 71 Multiple lesions are seen on the lips and gingival mucosa in herpetic stomatitis, a primary herpetic infection. The tongue is also extensively involved and covered with a greyish white membrane. A painful mouth, refusal to eat and fever are characteristic. Young children may require hospitalisation to ensure adequate fluid intake.

Fig. 72 There is a brown discoloration of the teeth due to severe hyperbilirubinaemia in the newborn period. This appearance is seen less often with the modern management of neonatal hyperbilirubinaemia.

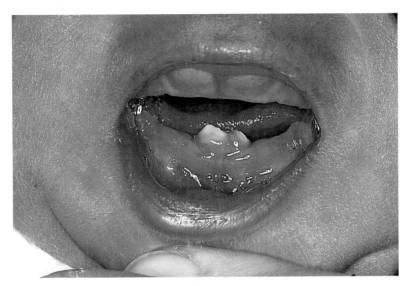

Fig. 73 Natal teeth

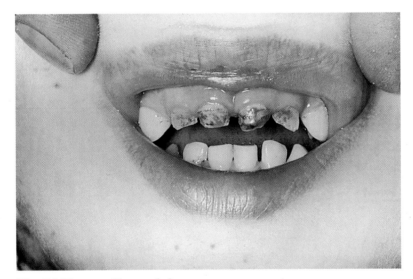

Fig. 74 Tetracycline staining

Fig. 73 Prematurely erupted teeth present at birth are termed natal teeth; teeth erupting in the first month are termed neonatal teeth. Usually two teeth are present in the position of the lower central incisor. Loose natal teeth should be extracted because of the risk of detachment and aspiration.

Fig. 74 This unsightly discoloration occurs in children given tetracyclines and in the primary teeth of children whose mothers were treated with tetracyclines during pregnancy. The condition is avoidable.

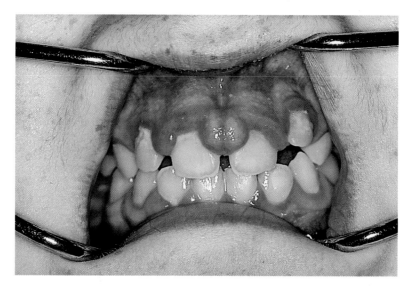

Fig. 75 Gum hypertrophy due to phenytoin

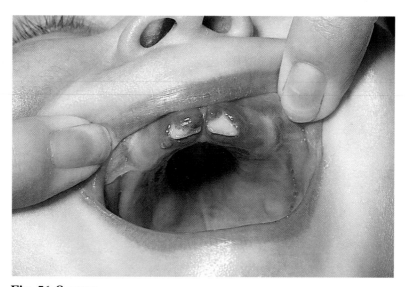

Fig. 76 Scurvy

Fig. 75 Gum hypertrophy due to phenytoin occurs in about 40% of patients taking this drug and is unrelated to dosage. The hypertrophy regresses over several months after phenytoin is discontinued, but dose reduction usually has little effect. This and other side-effects are seen less often nowadays, with the declining use of phenytoin in children.

Fig. 76 In vitamin C deficiency (scurvy), bleeding occurs in mucous membranes, soft tissues and skin, probably due to defective synthesis of collagen and other proteins which contribute to vascular support. Painful subperiosteal haemorrhages also occur.

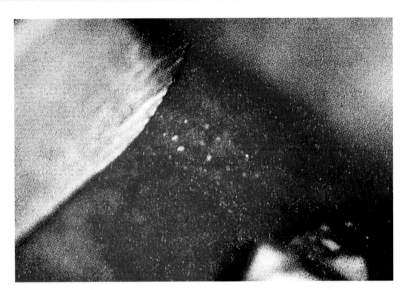

Fig. 77 Koplik spots

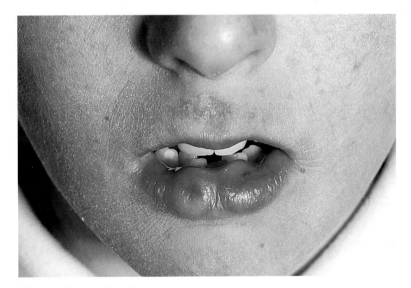

Fig. 78 Lower lip pits

Fig. 77 Koplik spots, tiny white dots on the buccal mucosa, are pathognomonic of measles and appear 1 or 2 days before the rash. They usually appear opposite the lower molars but can spread to other parts of the buccal mucosa. They disappear before the onset of the rash.

Fig. 78 Two pits set in small mounds are present in the lower lip. Several members of this boy's family had similar pits, suggesting autosomal dominant inheritance. Lower lip pits may be accompanied by a cleft lip, cleft palate and dental abnormalities in the autosomal dominant Van der Woude syndrome.

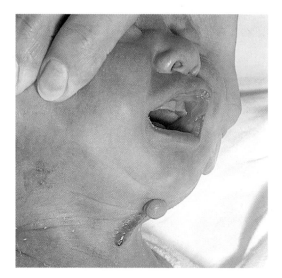

Fig. 79 Thyroglossal cyst

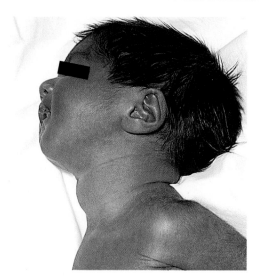

Fig. 80 Congenital goitre

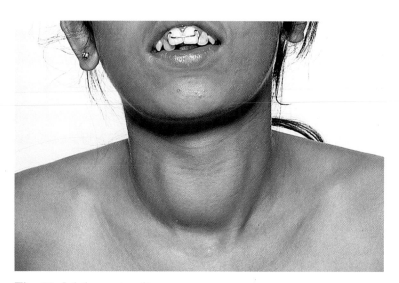

Fig. 81 Adolescent goitre

Fig. 79 A thyroglossal cyst presents as a cystic mass in the midline of the neck, most often in the region of the hyoid, and is usually asymptomatic. It occurs because of persistence of remnants of the thyroglossal duct. Treatment is by surgical excision.

Fig. 80 Diffuse enlargement of the thyroid is seen in this neonate whose head is held in extension. Very large goitres may cause respiratory distress in the newborn period. Congenital goitre may result from antithyroid drugs or iodine-containing preparations taken in pregnancy, defective thyroxine synthesis or iodine deficiency.

Fig. 81 This girl has diffuse enlargement of the thyroid gland. Colloid goitre is not uncommon in euthyroid adolescent girls but usually resolves spontaneously, although occasionally surgery should be considered on cosmetic grounds if the goitre is very large. Autoimmune thyroiditis should be excluded in all cases of adolescent goitre.

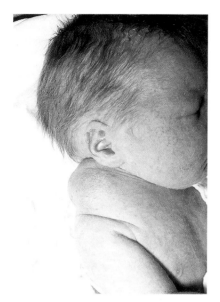

Fig. 82 Cystic hygroma

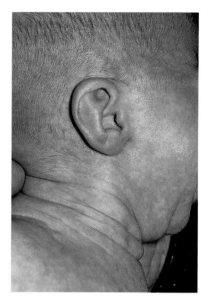

Fig. 83 Sternomastoid tumour

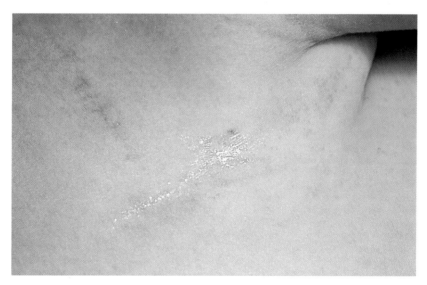

Fig. 84 Branchial cleft sinus

Fig. 82 This cystic hygroma is characterised by a large swelling on the side of the neck consisting of a mass of dilated lymphatic vessels. The face may also be involved. These masses are fluctuant and brilliantly transilluminate. Upper airways obstruction may occur in the neonatal period.

Fig. 83 There is swelling of the mid-portion of the right sternomastoid muscle. The 'tumour' represents an area of contracted fibrous tissue. If untreated, torticollis may result.

Fig. 84 In this case of branchial cleft sinus, a discharging sinus is present on the inferolateral aspect of the neck. Such sinuses and cysts result from the incomplete closure of the 1st, 2nd, 3rd or 4th branchial clefts during embryonic life. These lesions are usually unilateral and may open externally or drain into the pharynx. They are liable to recurrent infection and should be excised.

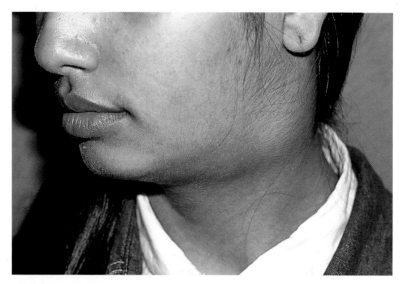

Fig. 85 Cervical lymphadenopathy

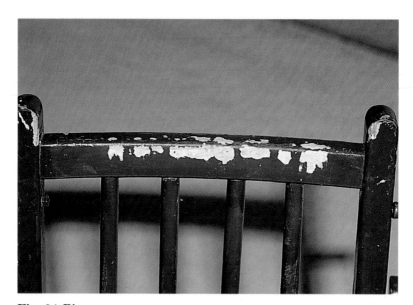

Fig. 86 Pica

Fig. 85 A mass is visible in the submandibular region of this girl's neck which proved to be due to tuberculous lymphadenitis. Tuberculous disease of the lymph nodes is usually unilateral, and the enlarged nodes are firm rather than hard and non-tender. These patients usually have few other symptoms and the chest X-ray is often normal. The differential diagnosis includes pyogenic infection, atypical mycobacterial infection and malignancy.

Fig. 86 This chair has received the attention of a child with pica (the eating of non-nutrient substances such as soil, plaster and flakes of paint). Pica is common in children with learning difficulties and may be a symptom of emotional deprivation. Iron deficiency is often present and the main dangers are lead poisoning and intestinal obstruction.

2 Chest and back

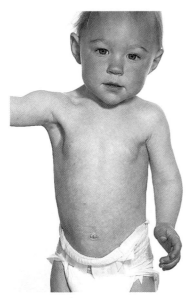

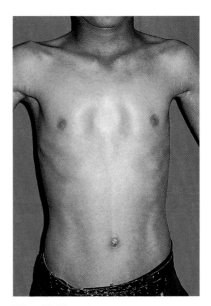

Fig. 87 Premature thelarche

Fig. 88 Pectus excavatum (funnel chest)

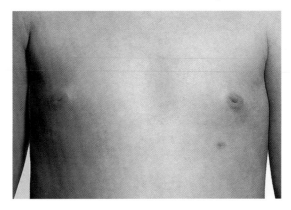

Fig. 89 Accessory nipple

Fig. 87 Bilateral breast development is seen in this toddler with premature thelarche who exhibited no other evidence of precocious puberty. Isolated breast development is a benign condition which occurs in children less than 3 years of age and is unaccompanied by other evidence of puberty or growth acceleration. Menarche occurs at the usual age. Pelvic ultrasound examination often shows a few ovarian cysts due to premature FSH secretion, but ovarian and uterine sizes are normal. Follow-up is necessary to ensure that other evidence of precocious puberty does not arise and that growth is normal.

Fig. 88 Pectus excavatum (funnel chest) is usually an isolated congenital abnormality but may be the result of chronic respiratory obstruction or, rarely, rickets. It is also seen in Turner syndrome and Marfan syndrome. Cardiorespiratory symptoms would be very unusual and surgical treatment is not indicated.

Fig. 89 Accessory nipple is a common minor anomaly occurring in both sexes. Supernumary nipples may occur anywhere along the embryological milk lines of the chest and abdomen. They may be mistaken for naevi. No treatment is required.

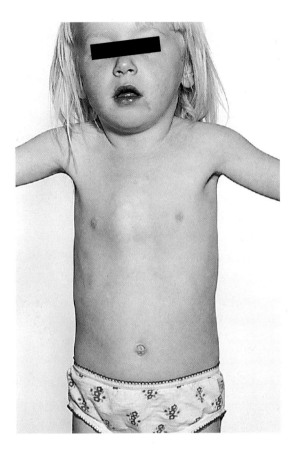

Fig. 90 Pectus carinatum (pigeon chest)

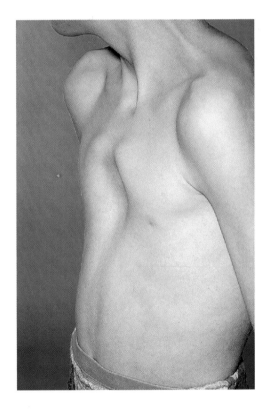

Fig. 91 Noonan syndrome

Fig. 90 In pectus carinatum (pigeon chest), the sternum is prominent and the thorax is slightly depressed laterally. Although this is a permanent deformity, it often becomes less noticeable after puberty and surgery should be avoided.

Fig. 91 The characteristic sternal abnormality in Noonan syndrome is pectus carinatum superiorly with pectus excavatum inferiorly. Webbing of the neck is also present. The other features of this syndrome are short stature, cardiac abnormalities (pulmonary stenosis or hypertrophic cardiomyopathy) and a characteristic facial appearance with hypertelorism, down-slanting palpebral fissures, ptosis and low set ears.

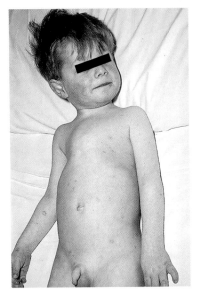

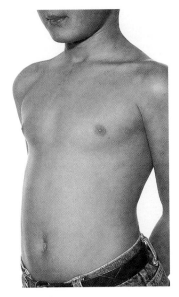

Fig. 92 Harrison's sulcus   **Fig. 93 Asthma**

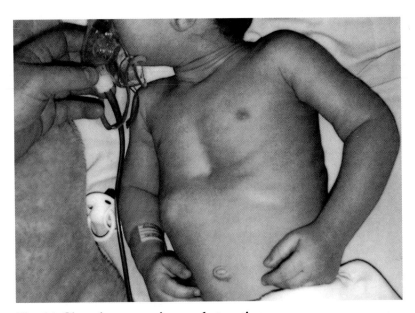

Fig. 94 Chronic upper airway obstruction

Fig. 92 In Harrison's sulcus, a horizontal depression is present along the lower part of the chest wall. This corresponds with the attachments of the diaphragm to the ribs. The condition is seen most often in chronic respiratory disease but may also occur in rickets.

Fig. 93 Inspection of chest shape is an important part of the assessment of the asthmatic child. This boy with poorly controlled asthma has an increased AP diameter of the chest due to hyperinflation.

Fig. 94 This child developed noisy breathing, sternal recession and hypoxemia during sleep. Her symptoms disappeared after removal of her tonsils and adenoids. Severe chronic upper airway obstruction may cause obstructive sleep apnoea, excessive daytime sleepiness and cor pulmonale. Grossly enlarged tonsils and adenoids are often present.

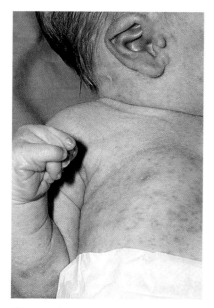

Fig. 95 Poland anomaly

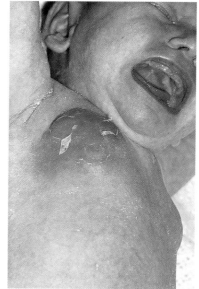

Fig. 96 Neonatal mastitis

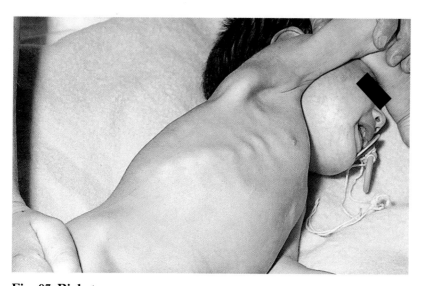

Fig. 97 Rickets

Fig. 95 Unilateral hypoplasia of the right pectoralis major muscle is seen. This accompanies deficiency of the distal part of the arm on the same side with syndactyly. Poland anomaly is sporadic and the aetiology is unknown. It is much more common in boys and the right side is most often affected.

Fig. 96 Neonatal breast enlargement is common but occasionally infection, usually due to *Staphylococcus aureus*, develops. This baby has redness, swelling and tenderness of the right breast. Treatment is with antibiotics, including an antistaphylococcal agent.

Fig. 97 In this case of rickets, swelling of the costochondral junctions on the right side of the chest is seen ('rachitic rosary').

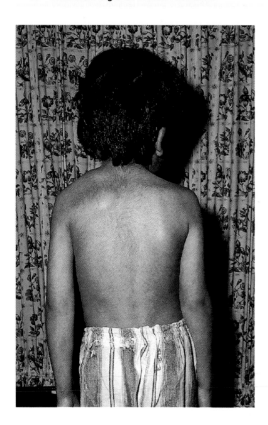

Fig. 98 Sprengel deformity

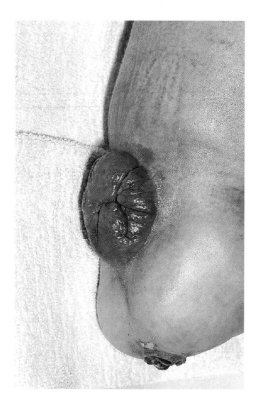

Fig. 99 Myelomeningocele

Fig. 98 The left scapula is small, abnormally high and medially rotated. The scapula is hypoplastic and attached muscles may be underdeveloped and weak. Failure of caudal migration, which normally occurs in the first trimester, is the cause of Sprengel deformity.

Fig. 99 There is a midline defect in the lumbar region through which protrudes a sac-like structure containing neural tissue and CSF. Such a defect is accompanied by neurological signs in the lower limbs and bladder and bowel dysfunction. Hydrocephalus often develops. Fortunately, neural tube defects have become less common in recent years.

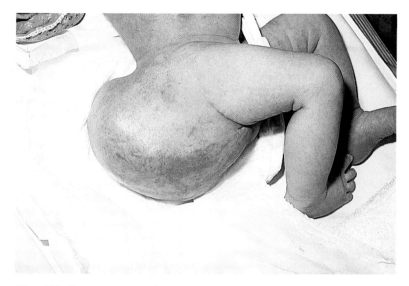

Fig. 100 **Sacrococcygeal teratoma**

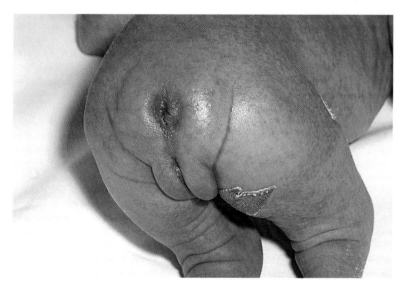

Fig. 101 **Sacral agenesis**

Fig. 100 There is a large midline mass arising from this baby's coccyx. Sacrococcygeal teratoma is the commonest tumour presenting in the neonatal period and contains tissue from all three germ areas. Most are benign and can often be completely excised. Malignant change becomes much more frequent by the age of 2 months.

Fig. 101 Weakness of the pelvic floor musculature is present in this baby with sacral agenesis. Developmental defects of the lower limbs are often present and there may be other associated congenital abnormalities, especially of the genitourinary and gastrointestinal tracts. There is a strong association with maternal diabetes.

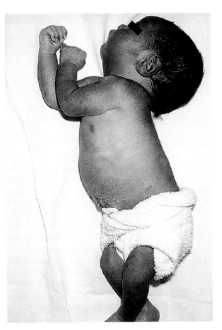

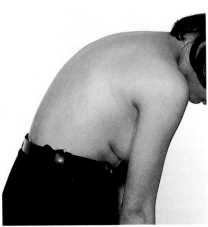

Fig. 102 Scheuermann kyphosis   **Fig. 103 Kernicterus**

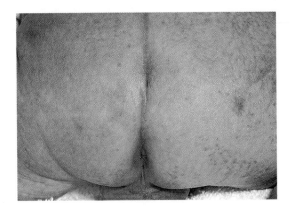

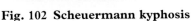

Fig. 104 Sacrococcygeal pit

Fig. 102 In Scheuermann kyphosis, increased kyphotic angulation is present on forward bending, which is due to an abnormality of ossification of the anterior vertebral bodies. The condition usually presents in adolescence with back pain. Radiologically, the vertebral bodies show irregularities of the anterior vertebral growth plates and wedging of adjacent vertebral bodies.

Fig. 103 Kernicterus is a neurological condition due to deposition of unconjugated bilirubin in brain cells. Fortunately, it is uncommon nowadays, thanks to modern management of rhesus incompatibility and hyperbilirubinaemia. This baby is showing an opisthotonic posture with neck retraction. The arms are inwardly rotated and the fists clenched. Other clinical features of this condition include lethargy, convulsions, bulging fontanelle and a high-pitched cry. Survivors often develop athetoid cerebral palsy, deafness and mental retardation.

Fig. 104 A blind ending sinus or pit is present in the midline intergluteal cleft over the sacrum. Sacrococcygeal pit is a common, benign asymptomatic finding in infants. However, congenital midline sinuses at a higher level are a portal of entry for bacteria and predispose to bacterial meningitis.

3 Abdomen and genitalia

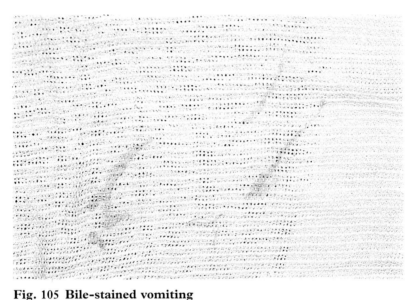

Fig. 105 Bile-stained vomiting

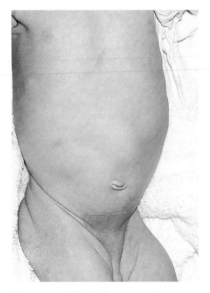

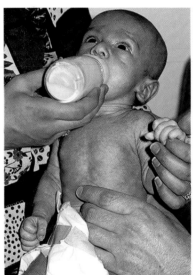

Fig. 106a Pyloric stenosis   **Fig. 106b Pyloric stenosis**

Fig. 105 Bile-stained vomiting should always suggest intestinal obstruction distal to the second part of the duodenum. (In this case, the baby was found to have malrotation and volvulus.) However, vomiting, if repeated, may eventually become bile-stained in the absence of obstruction if duodenal contents reflux into the stomach.

Fig. 106a–b (**a**) Visible peristalsis is seen in the epigastric region of this child who presented with projectile vomiting and weight loss. This sign with such a history is highly suggestive of pyloric stenosis. Palpation of a pyloric tumour, which waxes and wanes in consistency during feeding, confirms the diagnosis of pyloric stenosis. (**b**) Palpation is carried out with the left hand just lateral to the right rectus and below the liver edge. The tumour, which feels like an olive, is most easily palpated immediately after vomiting. Palpation is also easier if the stomach is relatively empty.

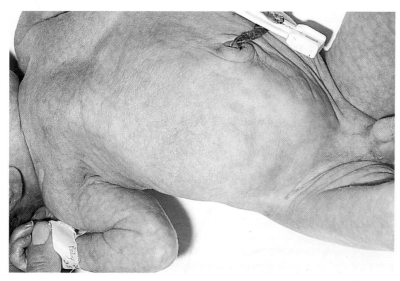

Fig. 107 Prune belly syndrome

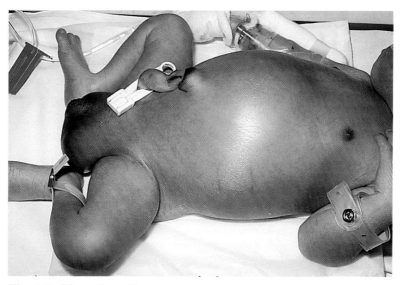

Fig. 108 Meconium ileus

Fig. 107 The wrinkled 'prune-like' appearance of the abdomen is due to deficiency of the abdominal wall muscles. Prune belly syndrome, which occurs almost exclusively in boys, is often accompanied by undescended testes and urinary tract abnormalities such as megacystis, grossly dilated ureters and hydronephrosis. Bowel malrotation and musculoskeletal and cardiac abnormalities may also be present.

Fig. 108 Abdominal distension and bilious vomiting in the neonate almost always indicate gastrointestinal obstruction. In meconium ileus, distension is present on the first day and meconium-filled loops are often palpable. X-ray shows a 'ground glass' appearance of air mixed with meconium. Approximately 20% of cystic fibrosis patients present with this condition.

Fig. 109 Cystic fibrosis

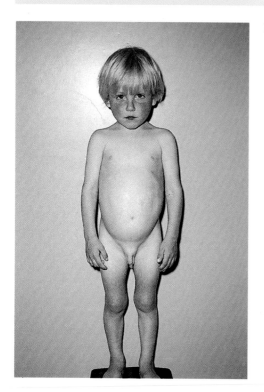

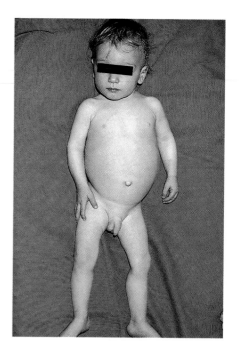

Fig. 110 Coeliac disease

Fig. 109 Abdominal distension and muscle wasting is present in this boy who presented with a history of frequent loose bulky stools and poor weight gain. Over 90% of cystic fibrosis patients have intestinal malabsorption due to pancreatic insufficiency. Diagnosis is based on two abnormal sweat chloride results on at least 100 mg of sweat.

Fig. 110 Coeliac disease classically presents in young children with chronic diarrhoea or large bulky stools, failure to thrive and abdominal distension. Affected children are often unhappy and irritable, and in contrast to children with cystic fibrosis often have a poor appetite. Presentation in older children is often more subtle – growth retardation rather than gastrointestinal symptoms may be the dominant clinical feature.

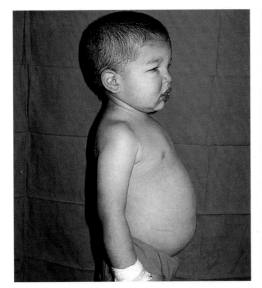

Fig. 111 Nephrotic syndrome

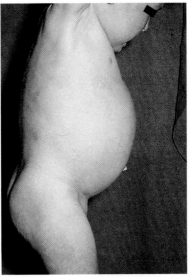

Fig. 112 Glycogen storage disease type I (von Gierke disease)

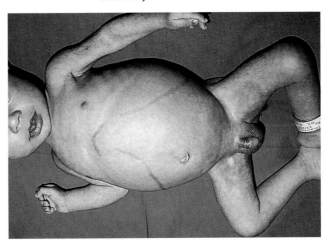

Fig. 113 Lipid storage disease

Fig. 111 Gross abdominal distension due to ascites is present in this boy who also has generalised oedema, heavy proteinuria and hypoproteinaemia. The majority of patients aged 2–6 years with this presentation have steroid-sensitive minimal change disease. Removal of ascitic fluid is not indicated unless peritonitis is suspected.

Fig. 112 In this child with glycogen storage disease type I (von Gierke disease), abdominal enlargement is due to gross hepatomegaly. The disease is due to absence or deficiency of glucose 6 phosphatase activity in liver, kidney and gastrointestinal mucosa. Children present at 3 or 4 months of age with hepatomegaly usually due to excessive accumulation of glycogen and hypoglycaemia. The spleen is not enlarged.

Fig. 113 Gross hepatosplenomegaly causing abdominal distension is present in this case of lipid storage disease. This patient had Wolman disease, which results in the storage of cholesterol and cholesteryl esters due to deficiency of acid lipase. Similar hepatosplenomegaly is seen in Niemann–Pick disease and Gaucher disease.

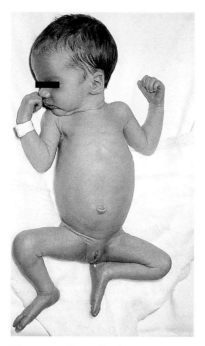

Fig. 114a Jaundice

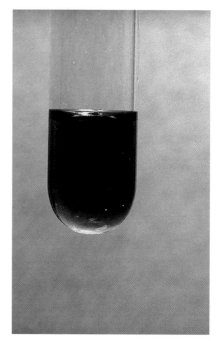

Fig. 114b Obstructive jaundice

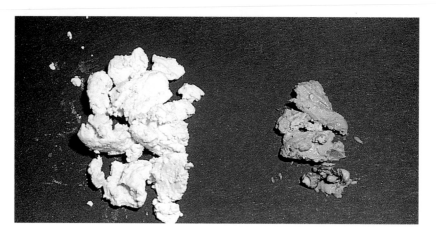

Fig. 115 Acholic stools

Fig. 114a–b (**a**) Jaundice is probably the commonest 'clinical sign' in paediatric practice, affecting up to 50% of normal term babies. Important points to remember are: (1) jaundice in the first 24 hours is likely to be due to blood group incompatibility; (2) jaundice appearing towards the end of the first week can be due to infection; and (3) in persistent jaundice, conjugated hyperbilirubinaemia should be excluded. (**b**) The passage of dark brown urine together with acholic or clay-coloured stools indicates either extrahepatic biliary obstruction or an intrahepatic process which inhibits bile flow.

Fig. 115 Very pale stools from an infant with biliary atresia are seen here beside normal stools. Conjugated hyperbilirubinaemia, dark urine, acholic stools and hepatomegaly occur in both biliary atresia and neonatal hepatitis. It is important to diagnose the former in the first 6 weeks of life if surgery is to be effective.

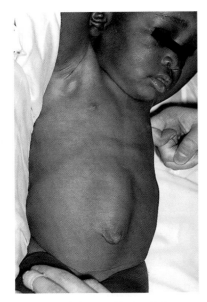

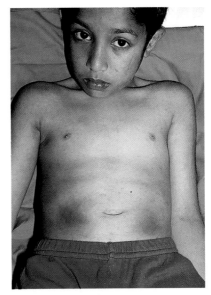

Fig. 116 Divarcation of the recti (diastasis recti)

Fig. 117 Thalassaemia

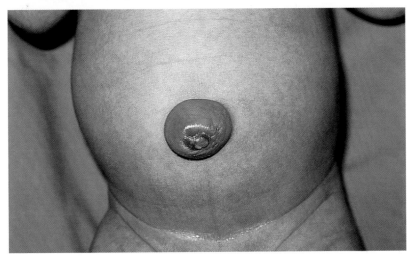

Fig. 118 Umbilical hernia

Fig. 116 A gap between the rectus muscles, most noticeable with crying, is a common harmless anomaly in neonates requiring only parental reassurance.

Fig. 117 Brown staining of the abdominal wall is present due to regular subcutaneous administration of the iron-chelating agent desferrioxamine in this transfusion-dependent thalassaemia patient. The absence of this sign is useful as it suggests poor compliance with treatment.

Fig. 118 A soft, skin-covered, easily reducible swelling is present at the umbilicus. Umbilical herniae are commoner in low birth weight babies and are more prominent during crying or straining. 'Strapping' is not effective and the great majority will spontaneously disappear by the end of the first year. Complications such as intestinal strangulation are very rare. A granuloma which was subsequently treated with silver nitrate is also present.

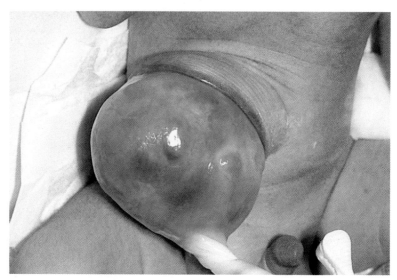

Fig. 119 Exomphalos

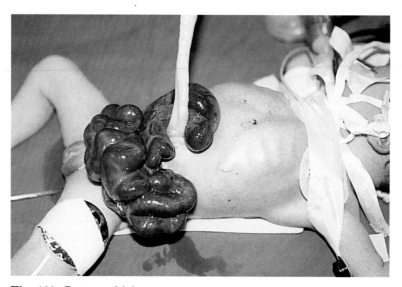

Fig. 120 Gastroschisis

Fig. 119 A large sac with a wide base containing abdominal contents covered by peritoneum is protruding through the umbilicus. Other congenital abnormalities may accompany exomphalos, e.g. congenital heart disease, chromosomal abnormalities, urinary tract anomalies and Beckwith–Wiedemann syndrome.

Fig. 120 In contrast to exomphalos (**Fig. 119**), the umbilical cord is normal in gastroschisis and loops of thickened bowel herniate through a small full-thickness defect in the anterior abdominal wall usually to the right of the umbilicus. There is no sac, and fluid loss can be significant.

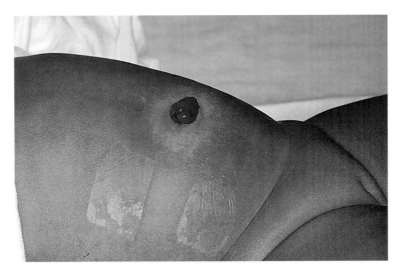

Fig. 121 Persistent vitello-intestinal duct

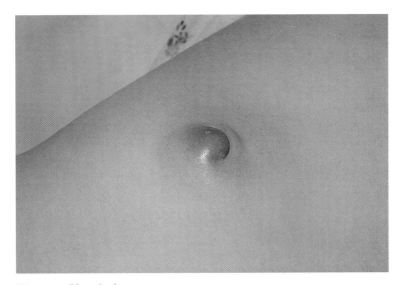

Fig. 122 Urachal cyst

Fig. 121 A small umbilical polyp covered by velvety red secreting mucosa is present due to persistence of the umbilical end of the vitello-intestinal duct. Persistence of the whole duct produces an intestinal fistula which discharges bowel content at the umbilicus. Persistence at the intestinal end of the duct results in a Meckel's diverticulum.

Fig. 122 The cystic swelling seen at the umbilicus is the result of persistence of the urachus, the primitive duct between the bladder and umbilicus. Patency of the urachus results in a urinary discharge at the umbilicus, but a cyst develops if the duct is closed above and below. Treatment is by excision.

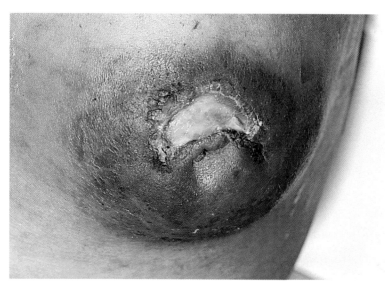

Fig. 123 Leucocyte adhesion deficiency

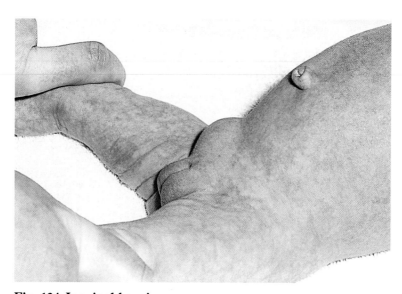

Fig. 124 Inguinal hernia

Fig. 123 Leucocyte adhesion deficiency is a rare disease due to deficiency of CD11/CD18 adhesion molecules which results in inability of phagocytes to migrate to sites of infection. Delayed umbilical cord separation and umbilical infection are common. There is often a persistent leucocytosis, and recurrent severe bacterial infection is common.

Fig. 124 Inguinal hernia typically appears as a reducible swelling in the groin which may only be apparent on crying. The vast majority of affected infants are male. Prematurity, chronic respiratory illness and ascites are predisposing features. Surgical treatment is always indicated to prevent strangulation.

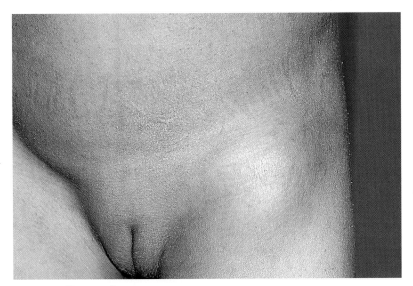

Fig. 125 Psoas abscess

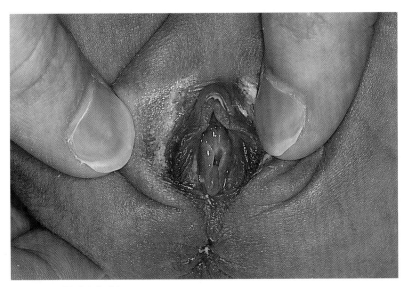

Fig. 126 Vulval skin tag

Fig. 125 A large swelling is present in the inguinal region and upper thigh. This may be accompanied by pyrexia, limp and hip pain. Psoas abscess may develop as an extension of infection from osteomyelitis of the spine, retroperitoneal appendicitis or Crohn's disease.

Fig. 126 A small vulval skin tag can be seen extending from the posterior hymen. This is a normal variant seen in infancy.

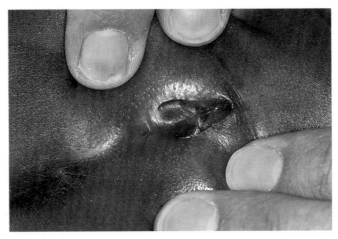

Fig. 127 Labial adhesions (labial agglutination)

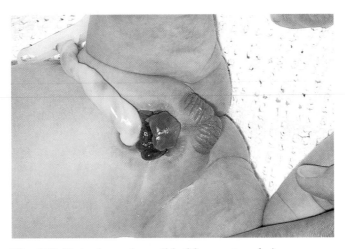

Fig. 128 Ectopia vesicae (bladder exstrophy)

Fig. 127 A bridge of tissue joining the labia minora can be seen extending upwards from the fourchette. Labial adhesions, which are common in girls under 5 years, may be asymptomatic or associated with local inflammation or urinary tract infection. Separation may be achieved by applying oestrogen cream.

Fig. 128 In this girl, the bladder is protruding from the abdominal wall with its mucosa exposed. There is downward displacement of the umbilicus and the pubic rami are separated. Ectopia vesicae is more common in boys, who also have epispadias. Girls also have duplication of the clitoris and wide separation of the labia.

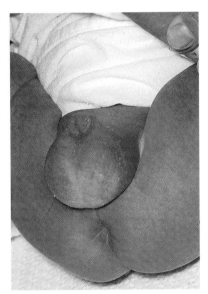

Fig. 129 **Bilateral hydroceles**

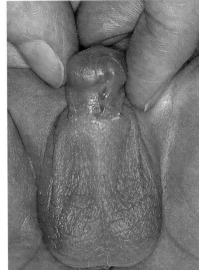

Fig. 130a **Hypospadias**

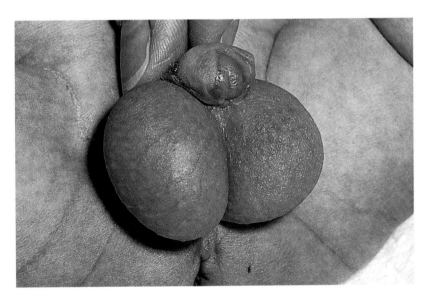

Fig. 130b **Hypospadias**

Fig. 129 Bilateral hydroceles present as fluid-filled scrotal swellings which transilluminate and cannot be reduced. Hydroceles should be distinguished from inguinal herniae and torsion of the testis. Most will resolve spontaneously.

Fig. 130a–b In hypospadias, the urethral meatus opens on the ventral surface of the penis just beneath the glans (**a**). The shaft of the penis curves ventrally (chordee). Severe hypospadias with cryptorchidism falls within the differential diagnosis of ambiguous genitalia and should be investigated. In some cases of hypospadias, particularly the more extensive cases, the scrotum is bifid (**b**), and may extend upwards to the base of the penis.

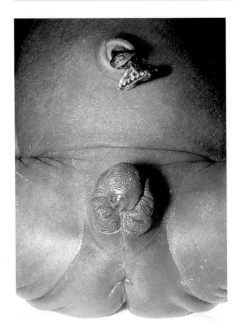

Fig. 131a Congenital adrenal hyperplasia

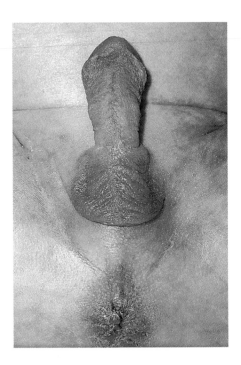

Fig. 131b Congenital adrenal hyperplasia

Fig. 131a–b (**a**) This patient with a female karyotype has ambiguous genitalia. There is a large phallus with fused rugiose labia. Congenital adrenal hyperplasia is the commonest cause of female pseudo-hermaphroditism. (**b**) Boys with this disorder who are not salt losers often escape detection in the first 2 weeks but present later with signs of inappropriate virilisation. The external genitalia may appear unremarkable at birth. This patient has penile enlargement but in contrast the testes appear small.

Fig. 132 Micropenis

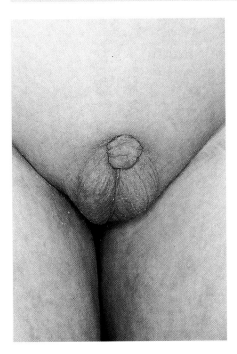

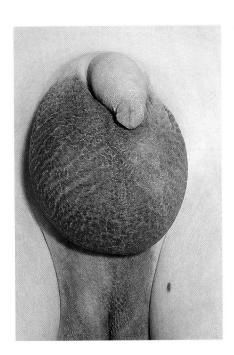

Fig. 133 Scrotal haematoma

Fig. 132 Often, an alleged small penis is of normal size (centile charts are available) but is enveloped in suprapubic fat. A true micropenis is 2.5 standard deviations below the mean length for age. Causes include hypothalamic/pituitary disorders, e.g. growth hormone deficiency and Prader–Willi syndrome, primary testicular disorders, e.g. Klinefelter's syndrome, and various dysmorphic syndromes.

Fig. 133 Scrotal haematoma may be due to violent trauma or, as in this case, a bleeding disorder. The patient was a haemophiliac who bled into his scrotum after a long bicycle ride. The haematoma subsided with factor VIII treatment.

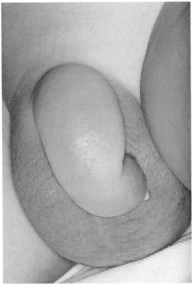

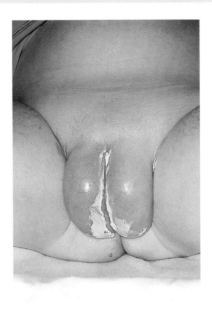

Fig. 134a Nephrotic syndrome   **Fig. 134b Nephrotic syndrome**

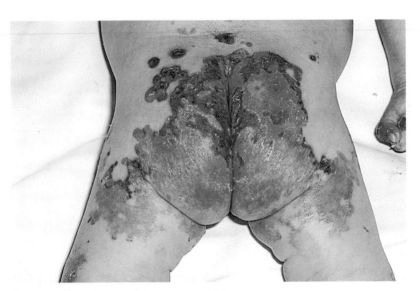

Fig. 135 Acrodermatitis enteropathica

Fig. 134a–b In cases of nephrotic syndrome, oedema often appears first in the scrotal and labial regions, as well as the periorbital regions. Oedema involving the external genitalia can be quite gross, uncomfortable and distressing.

Fig. 135 Acrodermatitis enteropathica is an autosomal recessive condition caused by defective zinc absorption from the gut. The rash, which typically occurs after weaning from breast to cow's milk, consists of an erythematous exudative eczematous eruption involving the perineal and perioral areas, hands, feet and face. Other features include chronic diarrhoea and hair loss.

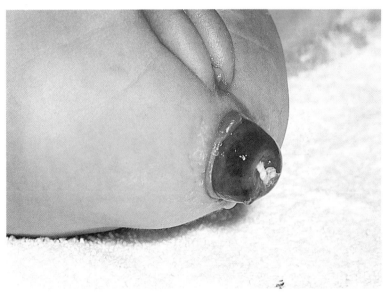

Fig. 136 Rectal prolapse

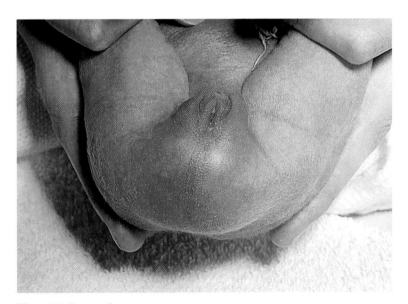

Fig. 137 Imperforate anus

Fig. 136 Rectal prolapse may occur because of weakness of the pelvic floor musculature (e.g. with spina bifida) or because of chronic diarrhoea or malnutrition. Cystic fibrosis should always be excluded. Treatment is by manual reduction. Submucosal injection of a sclerosant is effective in frequently recurring cases.

Fig. 137 Imperforate anus is obvious on routine examination of the newborn. Associated abnormalities, particularly of the urinary tract, are often present and should be excluded.

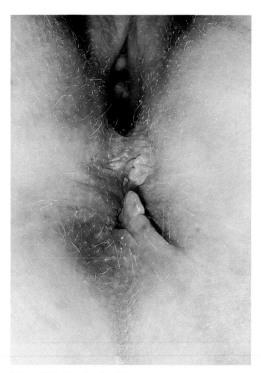

Fig. 138 Crohn's disease

Fig. 138 The perianal region is red and indurated, and a large skin tag and fissures are present. Perianal disease is quite common in Crohn's disease and perianal abscesses may also occur. Crohn's disease is often insidious in its presentation. Perianal inspection may provide a vital clue to the diagnosis in older children presenting with poor growth, anaemia, abdominal pain or diarrhoea.

4 Limbs

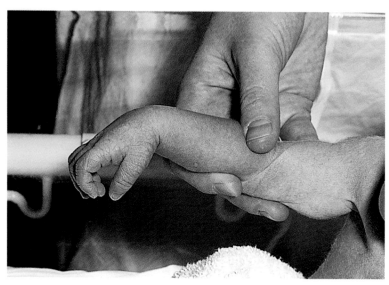

Fig. 139 Klumpke's paralysis

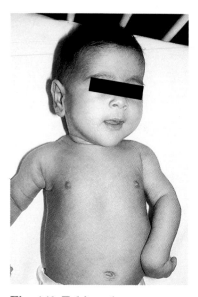

Fig. 140 Erb's palsy

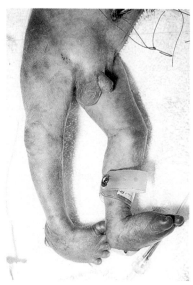

Fig. 141a Edward's syndrome (trisomy 18)

Fig. 139 Injury to the lower brachial plexus roots (C7, C8, T1) during delivery results in paralysis of the forearm flexors and extensors and of the intrinsic hand muscles (Klumpke's paralysis). The hand typically shows a claw-like posture. Involvement of the first thoracic root may also result in an accompanying Horner syndrome due to cervical sympathetic damage.

Fig. 140 Erb's palsy is the result of injury to the C5 and C6 brachial plexus nerve roots. This child's hand shows a typical 'waiter's tip' posture, with adduction and internal rotation of the arm and pronation of the forearm. This type of injury is usually the result of shoulder traction during delivery.

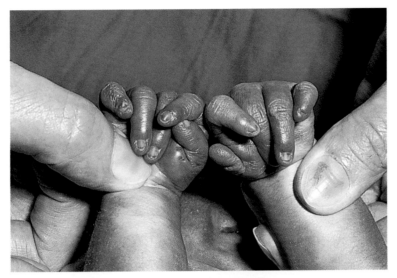

Fig. 141b Edward's syndrome (trisomy 18)

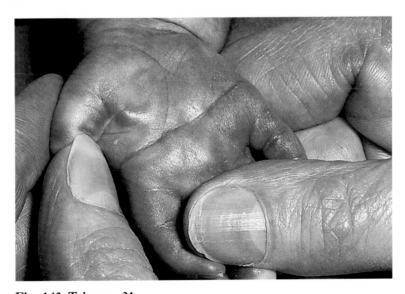

Fig. 142 Trisomy 21

Fig. 141a–b In cases of Edward's syndrome (trisomy 18), the feet (**a**, opposite) have a characteristic 'rocker-bottom' appearance. The hands are typically clenched, with index fingers overlapping third fingers (**b**). These babies also have a prominent occiput, low set ears, small mouth and micrognathia. About 90% will die in the first year of life because of cardiac or central nervous system abnormalities or respiratory infection.

Fig. 142 A single palmar crease is present and there is a wide gap between the thumb and index finger. Children with trisomy 21 characteristically have short broad hands with a short curving fifth finger. Single palmar crease is not peculiar to trisomy 21 and can occur in people with a normal karyotype.

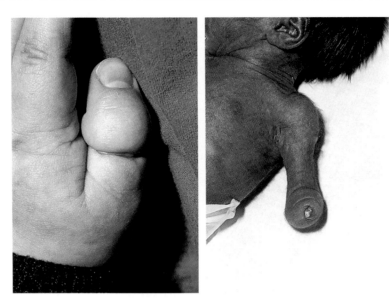

Fig. 143 Congenital ring constriction

Fig. 144a Congenital amputation

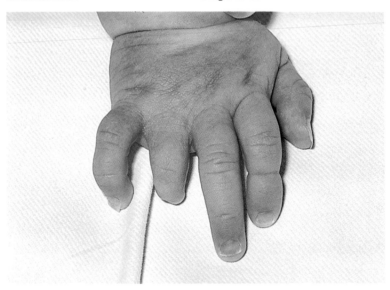

Fig. 144b Congenital amputation

Fig. 143 There is a constricting ring around the proximal phalanx of the thumb. This abnormality is probably due to an amniotic band being wrapped tightly around the digit. Localised oedema and amputation may also occur as a result of intrauterine constricting bands.

Fig. 144a–b (**a**) The left forearm was absent at birth as a result of intrauterine amputation. This is an example of disruption rather than malformation. In utero, the normally developed arm has become entangled in strands of amnion following amniotic rupture, resulting in constriction of the limb with subsequent amputation. (**b**) In this case, most of the fourth digit is missing, almost certainly as a result of an amniotic band being tightly wrapped around the digit in utero resulting in amputation.

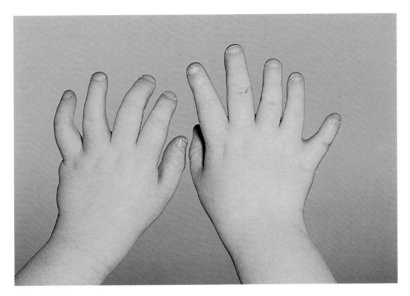

Fig. 145 Polydactyly

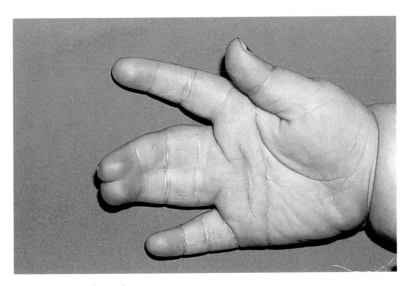

Fig. 146 Syndactyly

Fig. 145 Six digits are present in this patient's right hand. Polydactyly is often an isolated abnormality and can be familial but is found in a number of syndromes, e.g. Ellis–van Creveld syndrome, Carpenter syndrome and trisomy 13. In this particular case, the patient had the Laurence–Moon–Biedl syndrome. In addition to polydactyly, he had retinitis pigmentosa, obesity and hypogonadism.

Fig. 146 There is fusion of the soft tissues of the 3rd and 4th fingers (the commonest digits to be involved). Syndactyly is a congenital abnormality which varies in severity, and fusion of the bones can also occur. Syndactyly of the toes may also be present. The condition may occur in isolation or as part of a syndrome, e.g. Apert syndrome, Carpenter syndrome, Holt–Oram syndrome.

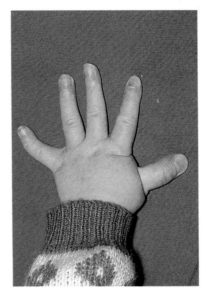

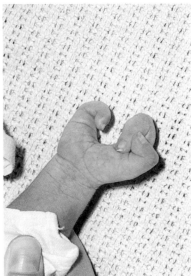

Fig. 147 Clinodactyly　　　　　**Fig. 148a Ectrodactyly**

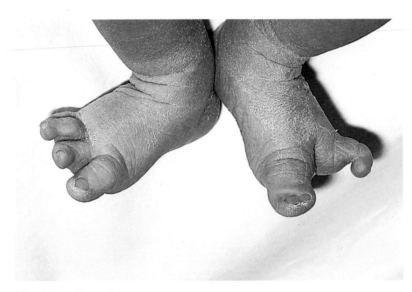

Fig. 148b Ectrodactyly

Fig. 147 In this case of clinodactyly, there is incurving of the 5th finger. This is occasionally seen as an isolated anomaly but is also a feature of a number of syndromes, the best known of which are Russell Silver syndrome and trisomy 21.

Fig. 148a–b In this case of ectrodactyly, there is 'splitting' of the hand and left foot, resulting in missing digits and V-shaped clefts. These abnormalities have sometimes been referred to as 'lobster claw' hands and feet. Other congenital abnormalities may be present, in particular cleft lip, cleft palate and ectodermal dysplasia. The combination of ectrodactyly, ectodermal dysplasia and clefting is referred to as the EEC syndrome and is inherited as an autosomal dominant disorder.

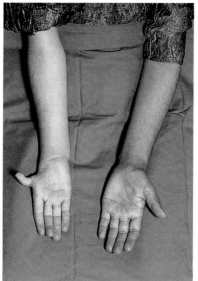

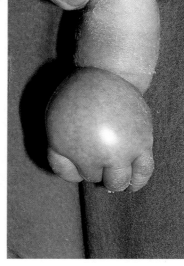

Fig. 149 Holt–Oram syndrome (cardiac limb syndrome)

Fig. 150a Turner syndrome

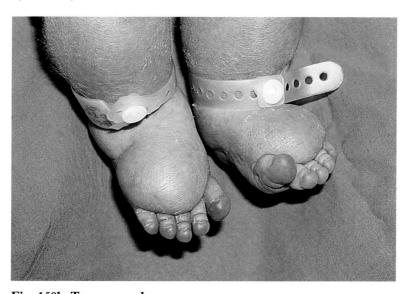

Fig. 150b Turner syndrome

Fig. 149 The right hand is small and the right thumb hypoplastic in this girl with Holt–Oram syndrome who also has an atrial septal defect. Different types of upper limb defect are seen in this syndrome, ranging from phocomelia to hypoplasia of the thumb. Defects may occur in all or any of the upper limb bones. Atrial septal defect and ventricular septal defect are the commonest cardiac defects.

Fig. 150a–b Although not exclusive to Turner syndrome, marked swelling of the dorsa of the hands and feet in the newborn is an indication for chromosome analysis. In Turner syndrome the nails are often hypoplastic. The swelling is due to disordered lymphatic drainage and the lymphoedema tends to regress afterwards. Occasionally, a tendency to develop intermittent oedema persists.

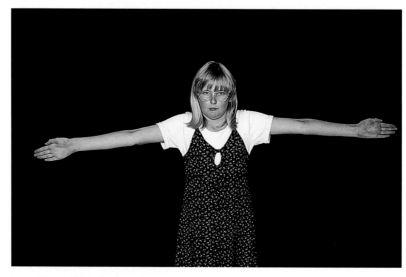

Fig. 151a Marfan syndrome

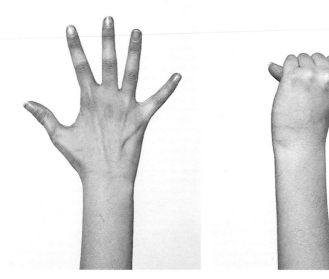

Fig. 151b Marfan syndrome   **Fig. 151c Marfan syndrome**

Fig. 151a–e (**a**) This patient's arm span exceeded her height by 4 cm. This is characteristic of Marfan syndrome. Normally, height just exceeds arm span. (**b**) This patient has long thin fingers (arachnodactyly). Typically, patients with Marfan syndrome are tall with long thin extremities and have joint hypermobility, anterior chest deformity and upward lens displacement. Cardiovascular problems include mitral regurgitation, aortic regurgitation and aortic dissection. (**c**) The same patient as in (b) is demonstrating Steinberg's sign in which the thumb, when opposed across the palm, extends beyond the ulnar border of the palm. (**d,e,** opposite) The diagnosis is more difficult to make in early infancy than in later childhood, but even at this age long thin hands and feet and arachnodactyly can be seen.

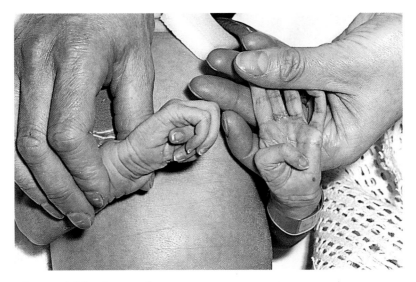

Fig. 151d Marfan syndrome

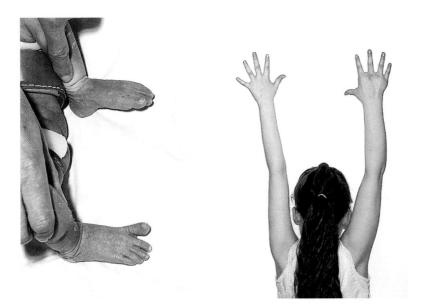

Fig. 151e Marfan syndrome   **Fig. 152 Hemihypertrophy**

Fig. 152 This child has an obvious enlargement of the right arm. Most cases of hemihypertrophy are idiopathic, although occasionally other abnormalities may be present. In particular, the increased incidence of Wilms' tumour should be remembered.

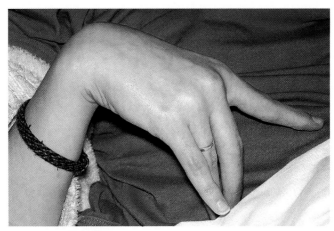

Fig. 153a Tetany

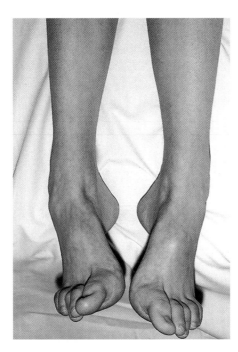

Fig. 153b Tetany

Fig. 153a–b (**a**) The typical hand posture of a carpopedal spasm is shown, with flexion of the wrist, extension of the fingers and adduction of the thumb over the palm (main d'accoucheur). In latent tetany, a spasm may be induced with a blood pressure cuff on the arm inflated above the systolic blood pressure for 3 or 4 minutes (Trousseau's sign). (**b**) Carpopedal spasm is seen at the ankles in the same patient as in (a). The feet are extended and adducted. Patients may also have sensory features such as paraesthesia of the hands and feet. Tetany results from a reduction in either ionised calcium or magnesium levels or from alkalosis.

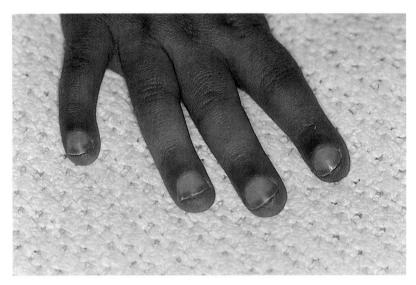

Fig. 154 **Finger clubbing**

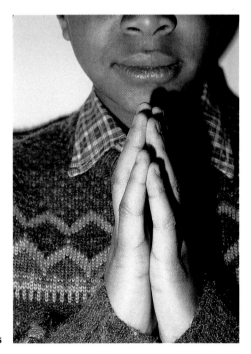

Fig. 155 **Diabetes mellitus**

Fig. 154 Swelling of the ends of the fingers is present in this child with congenital cyanotic heart disease. In clubbing, the nails become curved, both longitudinally and transversely. The earliest sign of clubbing is loss of the angle between the nail bed and soft tissue of the finger. Clubbing is rarely seen in the first year of life. It also occurs in chronic pulmonary disease, bowel disease and liver disease.

Fig. 155 Limited extension of the fingers is demonstrated by this boy with long-standing diabetes mellitus. Limited joint mobility may be associated with the early development of other diabetic complications such as nephropathy and retinopathy, although this has been disputed.

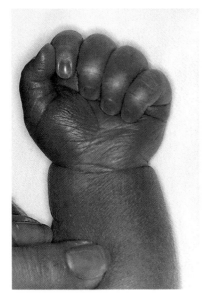

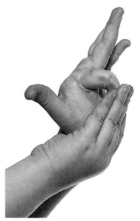

Fig. 156 Cold injury   **Fig. 157a Ehlers–Danlos syndrome**

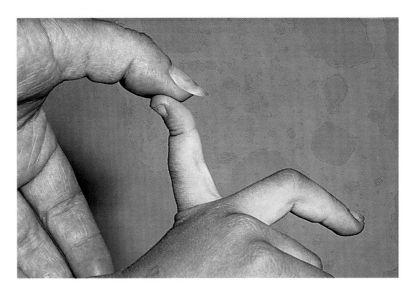

Fig. 157b Ehlers–Danlos syndrome

Fig. 156 The peripheries of this baby are cold and red due to low environmental temperature and inadequate clothing. Cold injury is still seen in the UK during the winter months.

Fig. 157a–d Ehlers–Danlos syndrome is characterised by hyperextensible skin, connective tissue fragility and hypermobile joints. This patient is able to hyperextend her fingers (**a**), hyperextend her terminal phalanges (**b**) and proximate her thumb to her forearm (**c**). Joint hypermobility in this

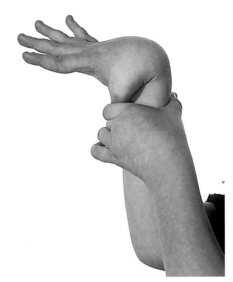

Fig. 157c Ehlers–Danlos syndrome

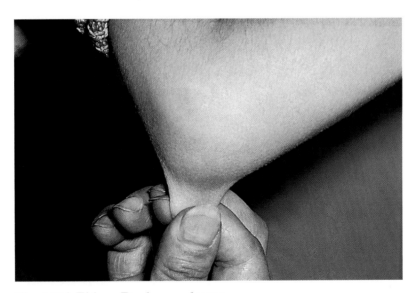

Fig. 157d Ehlers–Danlos syndrome

condition is associated with an increased incidence of congenital dislocation of the hip, frequent muscular aches and pains, joint sprains and an increased tendency to joint dislocation. Typical skin hyperextensibility is demonstrated at this second patient's elbow (**d**). When released, the stretched skin will resume its original position. In some patients, the skin stretching can be very impressive, while in others it is relatively minor. The skin is also characteristically fragile, splitting on minor trauma, healing slowly and then forming characteristic thin scars.

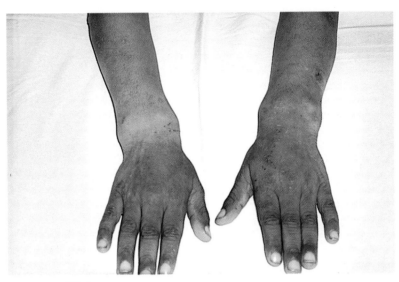

Fig. 158a Rickets

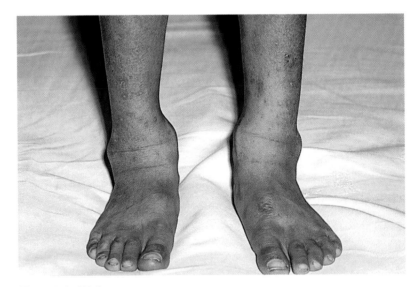

Fig. 158b Rickets

Fig. 158a–c (a,b) There is obvious epiphyseal enlargement of the wrists and ankles of this child with florid rickets. This disease is seen rarely in industrialised societies today, but is occasionally seen in immigrant children partly due to inadequate exposure to sunlight. (**c**, opposite) Bowing of the legs (genu varum) is seen in this child with nutritional rickets.

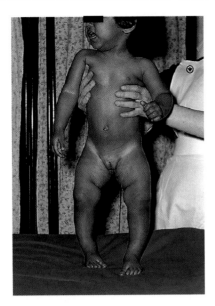

Fig. 158c Rickets

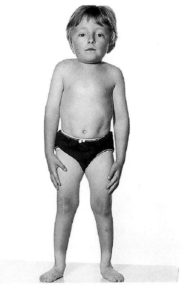

Fig. 159a Osteogenesis imperfecta type 3

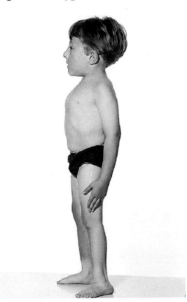

Fig. 159b Osteogenesis imperfecta type 3

Fig. 159a–b This 5-year-old girl has a history of multiple fractures, including antenatal fractures. She has marked short stature, chest deformity and a characteristic triangular appearance of the head. Her lower limb deformities have been largely corrected by orthopaedic surgery. Type III osteogenesis imperfecta is inherited as an autosomal recessive. The sclera are usually white, whereas the sclera in the less severe but more common type 1 osteogenesis imperfecta are often blue.

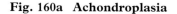

Fig. 160a   Achondroplasia

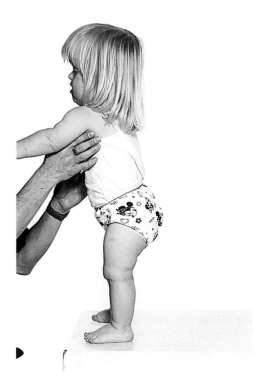

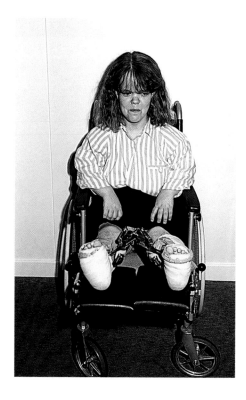

Fig. 160b Achondroplasia

Fig. 160a–b (**a**) This girl with short stature has short limbs, an increased head circumference with a prominent forehead and mid-facial hypoplasia with a flat nasal bridge. Most of the limb shortening occurs in the proximal limb segments. Lumbar lordosis develops and, quite often, spinal complications occur, resulting in cord or root compression. Hydrocephalus due to a narrow foramen magnum is a further complication. (**b**) This girl with achondroplasia has short upper limbs and a typical facial appearance with low nasal bridge and prominent forehead. She has had recent surgery to straighten and lengthen her lower limbs. Inheritance of achondroplasia is autosomal dominant, although the majority of cases represent new mutations. There is an association with older paternal age.

Fig. 161a Hypochondroplasia

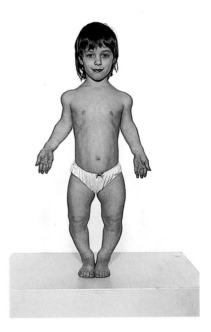

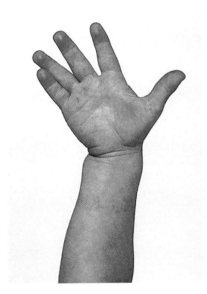

Fig. 161b Hypochondroplasia

Fig. 161a–b Hypochondroplasia, an autosomal dominant condition which presents as short-limbed short stature, has some overlap with achondroplasia. There is considerable shortening of the upper and lower limbs with marked bowing of the legs (**a**), but in contrast to achondroplasia, the head size and facial features are normal. Radiologically the long bones are short and widened with flared metaphyses. Short digits and wide hands (**b**) are characteristic of both achondroplasia and hypochondroplasia. The hand often resembles a trident consisting of the thumb, the 2nd and 3rd fingers, and the 4th and 5th fingers.

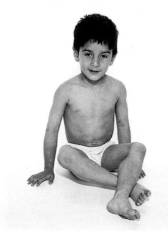

Fig. 162a Duchenne muscular dystrophy

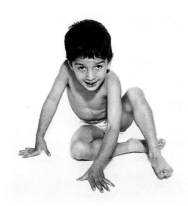

Fig. 162b Duchenne muscular dystrophy

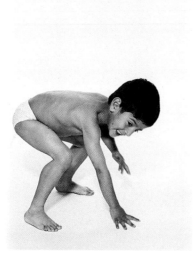

Fig. 162c Duchenne muscular dystrophy

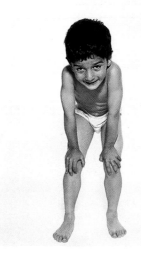

Fig. 162d Duchenne muscular dystrophy

Fig. 162a–e (**a–d**) This boy with Duchenne muscular dystrophy is showing Gower's sign, which is an indication of proximal muscle weakness in the lower limbs. This sign is observed by asking the child to rise from a sitting position. As a result of proximal weakness, he has to use his hands to 'climb up' the legs in order to stand upright. This sign is usually present by the age of 3–4 years. (**e**, opposite) Enlargement of the calves (pseudohypertrophy) due to fat infiltration of muscle and collagen proliferation is a classical feature of this condition. Other muscles, including those of the tongue, may be affected.

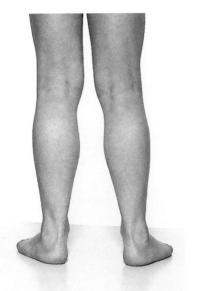

Fig. 162e Duchenne muscular dystrophy

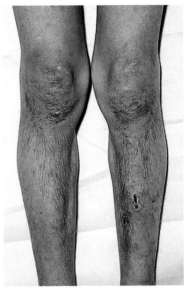

Fig. 163a Congenital insensitivity to pain

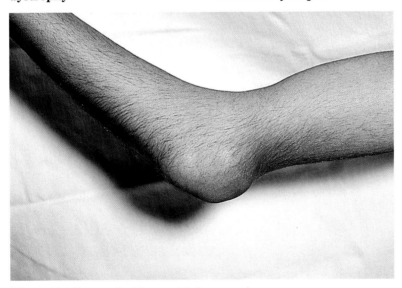

Fig. 163b Congenital insensitivity to pain

Fig. 163a–b Evidence of repeated injuries to the lower limbs is seen (**a**) due to lack of pain perception in this boy who was otherwise neurologically normal. The same patient has a grossly abnormal elbow joint (Charcot's joint) (**b**). There has been massive joint destruction secondary to repeated injury associated with lack of pain perception.

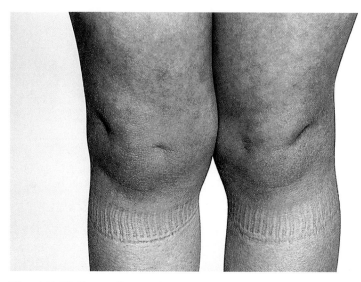

Fig. 164 Nail–patella syndrome

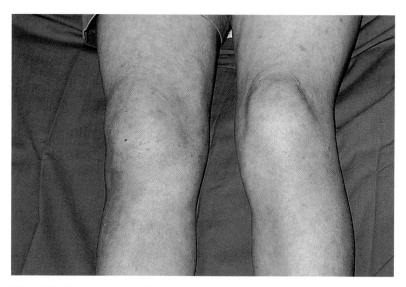

Fig. 165 Reactive arthritis

Fig. 164 In this case of nail–patella syndrome, the left patella is noticeably smaller than the right and is hypoplastic. The nails are also small and hypoplastic in this autosomal dominant disorder. Other skeletal abnormalities may be present, and renal disease, which may progress to renal failure, is present in 30–40% of patients.

Fig. 165 This girl developed a sterile effusion of the right knee joint following a throat infection. The swelling settled spontaneously within a few weeks. Transient aseptic arthritis may be due to viral infections (e.g. rubella, Epstein–Barr virus, parvovirus) and may occur after gastrointestinal, meningococcal, *Haemophilus* or streptococcal infection.

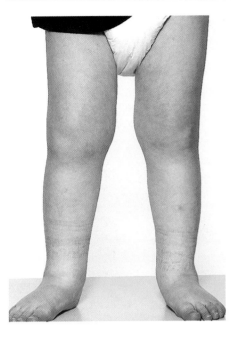

Fig. 166 Juvenile chronic arthritis

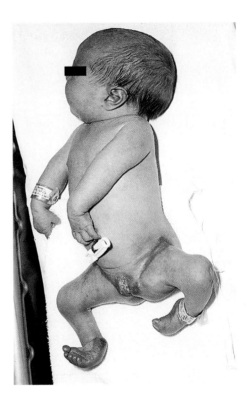

Fig. 167 Arthrogryposis

Fig. 166 The right knee joint is swollen and painful in this boy with antinuclear factor positive pauciarticular (fewer than five joints) juvenile chronic arthritis (JCA). Pauciarticular disease is the commonest JCA subgroup. Such children require regular slit lamp examination by an ophthalmologist to detect chronic uveitis.

Fig. 167 This baby with arthrogryposis had multiple joint contractures at birth. The shoulders are held in adduction and internal rotation, the elbows are held in extension and the wrists are fixed in flexion. Fixed flexion deformities are present at the knees and ankles. The muscles and tissues around these joints are hypoplastic or fibrotic. This syndrome is the end result of a number of neuropathic or myopathic conditions.

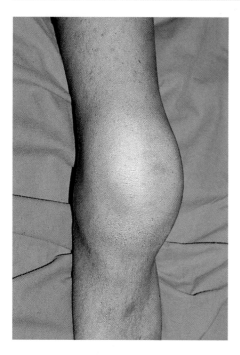

Fig. 168 Haemarthrosis

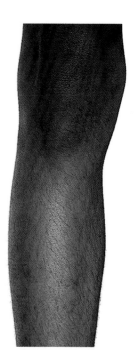

Fig. 169 Osgood–Schlatter disease

Fig. 168 Bleeding into large joints occurring spontaneously or following minor trauma is the hallmark of severe haemophilia. The swollen joint is warm and painful, and movement is limited. Degenerative changes occur with repeated haemorrhage and early treatment with factor VIII is essential. Bleeding often recurs in the same joint – 'the target joint'.

Fig. 169 In Osgood–Schlatter disease, there is a painful tender swelling of the tibial tuberosity. This inflammatory condition is common in childhood or adolescence, especially in athletic children. The condition is benign and self-limiting. Treatment consists of avoiding activities which involve quadriceps contraction.

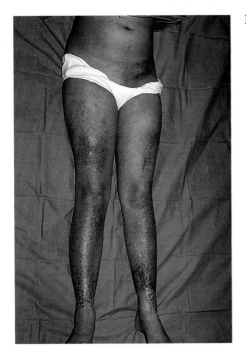

Fig. 170a Hyperimmunoglobulin E syndrome

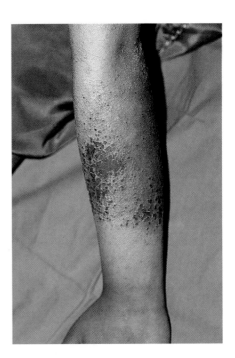

Fig. 170b Hyperimmunoglobulin E syndrome

Fig. 170a–b This girl with hyperimmunoglobulin E syndrome has a chronic pruritic dermatitis involving her arms and legs. The distribution is different to that of typical atopic eczema, which characteristically involves the flexures. In addition, she has subcutaneous abscesses involving the left inguinal region and anterior aspects of both thighs. Typically for this condition, symptoms of inflammation such as pain, redness and local heat are absent. Pus containing *Staphylococcus aureus* was drained from the abscesses. The main features of this syndrome are chronic dermatitis, recurrent staphylococcal abscesses, pneumonia often with pneumatoceles, and extremely high serum IgE levels.

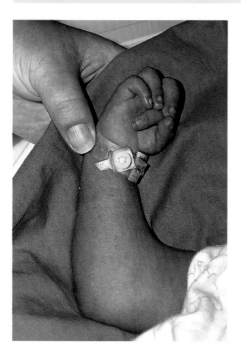

**Fig. 171a Multiple pterygium syndrome
(Escobar syndrome)**

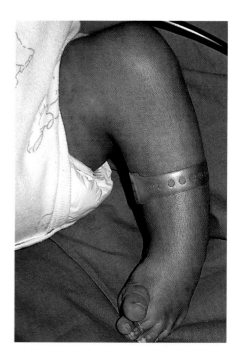

**Fig. 171b Multiple pterygium syndrome
(Escobar syndrome)**

Fig. 171a–b In multiple pterygium syndrome (Escobar syndrome), tight folds of tissue (pterygia) are present at the antecubital and popliteal fossae. There is also irreducible flexion of the fingers (camptodactyly) (**a**) and equinovarus deformity of the foot (**b**). Pterygia involving the neck and axillae also occur in this autosomal recessive disorder. Patients also have short stature and a characteristic facies with downward slant to the eyes, ptosis, hypertelorism and micrognathia. Intelligence is normal.

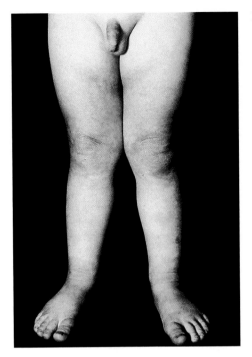

Fig. 172 Genu valgum (knock-knees)

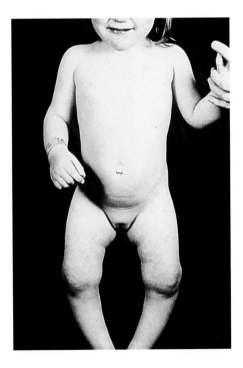

Fig. 173 Genu varum (bow legs)

Fig. 172 Genu valgum (knock-knees) is common in children aged 2–6 years and is most often physiological. Pathological causes, which are relatively uncommon, include rickets, skeletal dysplasias and neurological disorders. Almost all physiological cases resolve spontaneously. The distance between medial malleoli can be measured to monitor progress, a separation of more than 9 or 10 cm being an indication for orthopaedic referral.

Fig. 173 Genu varum is, like genu valgum, most often physiological. It is a common finding in infants and toddlers, but spontaneous resolution with normal growth and development nearly always occurs. Pathological causes of genu varum include Blount disease (tibia vara), skeletal dysplasias and rickets.

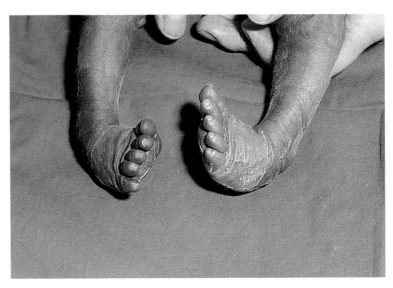

Fig. 174 Talipes equinovarus (club foot)

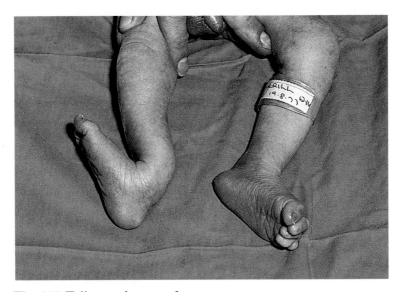

Fig. 175 Talipes calcaneovalgus

Fig. 174 In talipes equinovarus (club foot), both feet show plantarflexion of the hindfoot (equinus), with inversion of the ankles and adduction of the forefoot. This common congenital abnormality affects boys more than girls. Most cases are idiopathic although some are secondary to neuro-muscular disorders such as myelomeningocele. Management of this case is likely to involve serial plaster casts and perhaps surgery.

Fig. 175 There is excessive dorsiflexion of the right ankle with eversion of the foot. Talipes calcaneovalgus, which is present at birth, is often related to the intrauterine position of the foot and usually improves spontaneously by the age of 2 years. Congenital vertical talus and neurological abnormalities should be considered in the differential diagnosis.

Fig. 176 Pes cavus

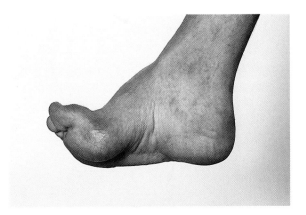

Fig. 177 Congenital absence of the fibula

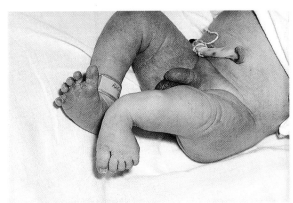

Fig. 178 Haematoma of the foot

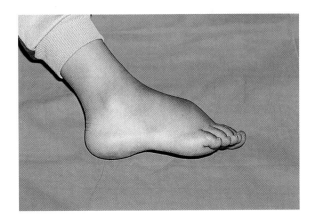

Fig. 176 In pes cavus, there is gross exaggeration of the medial longitudinal arch of the foot. This deformity may occur in isolation, but neurological disease such as Friedreich's ataxia or Charcot–Marie–Tooth disease should be excluded.

Fig. 177 There is gross bowing and distortion of the right lower limb due to congenital absence of the fibula. The lateral part of the foot may also be missing in this condition, which is also referred to as congenital fibular hemimelia. Surgical reconstruction is very difficult.

Fig. 178 There is swelling of the dorsum of the foot due to a haematoma which occurred following minimal trauma. Bleeding into the joints and haematoma characteristically occur in children with factor VIII and factor IX deficiency.

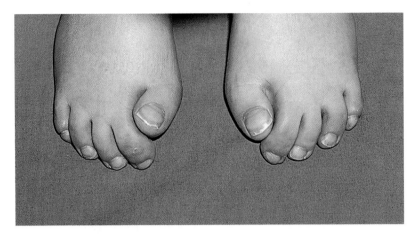

Fig. 179a Myositis ossificans

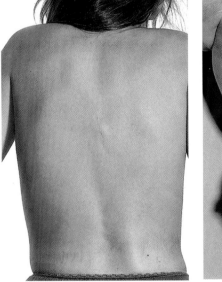

Fig. 179b Myositis ossificans

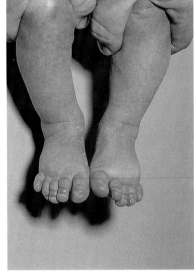

Fig. 180 Milroy's disease

Fig. 179a–b Myositis ossificans is a rare autosomal dominant condition characterised by progressive ectopic ossification and abnormal big toes. In this patient, the big toes are characteristically short and deviated laterally (**a**). Ectopic ossification commonly begins in the neck or dorsal spinal region and may be precipitated by trauma, biopsy of the lumps and intramuscular injection. This patient shows a scar (**b**) from a biopsy site (biopsies should be avoided if possible). Progressive limitation of movement and physical handicap occur due to ossification of joint capsules and voluntary muscle.

Fig. 180 The right leg is swollen because of lymphoedema. Milroy's disease, which may be present at birth or may develop later, is due to a congenital abnormality of the lower limb lymphatic channels. As opposed to oedema, pitting may not be present in lymphoedema.

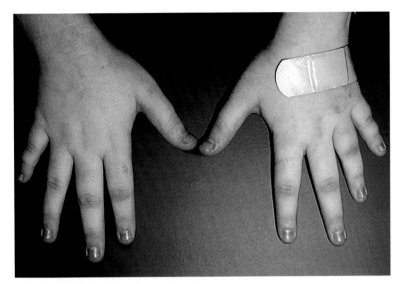

Fig. 181a Pseudohypoparathyroidism

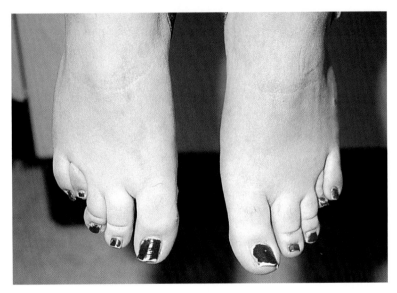

Fig. 181b Pseudohypoparathyroidism

Fig. 181a–b (**a**) This patient with pseudohypoparathyroidism has shortening of the metacarpals due to premature fusion of the epiphyses. The other features of this syndrome are hypocalcaemia and hyperphosphataemia due to end organ resistance to PTH, mental retardation, short stature, obesity and a round face. (**b**) In addition to changes affecting the metacarpals and metatarsals, the phalanges may also be involved. Very small fourth toes are seen in this patient.

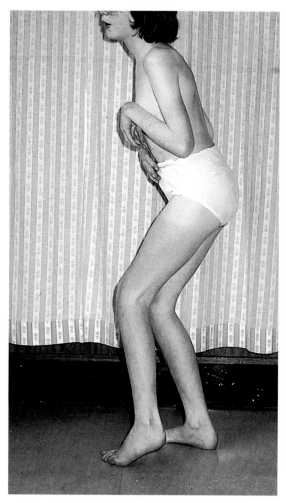

Fig. 182 Hemiplegia

Fig. 182 The characteristic posture of a child with a severe left hemiplegia is shown. The affected leg is shorter and the child walks on tip-toes due to spasticity and tightening of the left Achilles tendon. The left arm is flexed at the wrist and elbow and is adducted. In hemiplegia, the arm is often more severely affected than the leg.

5 Skin

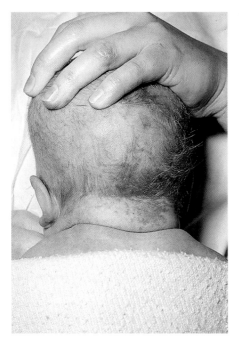

Fig. 183a Salmon patch haemangioma

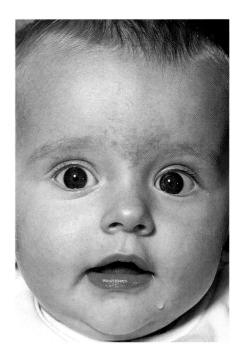

Fig. 183b Salmon patch haemangioma

Fig. 183a–b Salmon patch haemangiomata – pink macular areas involving the forehead, glabella, upper eyelids and back of the neck – are common in neonates. These lesions fade during the first year, with the exception of the neck lesion which is permanent but is eventually covered by hair. These lesions are also referred to as 'stork marks'.

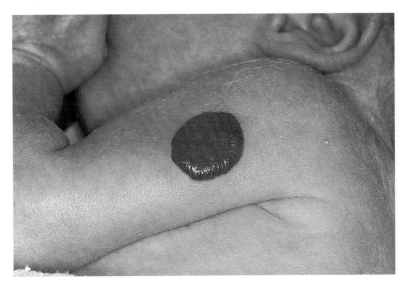

Fig. 184 Strawberry marks

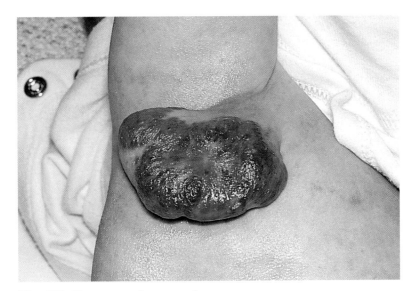

Fig. 185 Cavernous haemangioma

Fig. 184 Strawberry marks (superficial haemangiomata) are bright red well-demarcated lesions. They are not usually present at birth but appear in the first month on any part of the body. They grow rapidly during the first year, become static and then involute completely, usually by the age of 5 years.

Fig. 185 Cavernous haemangiomata are similar to superficial haemangiomata, only deeper. They also tend to involute spontaneously. Complications are rare, but they include ulceration, haemorrhage and infection. They may occur at 'difficult' sites, such as the axilla in this patient.

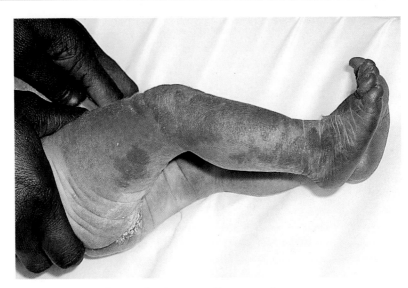

Fig. 186 Port wine stain (naevus flammeus)

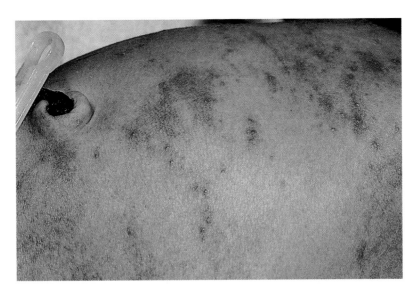

Fig. 187 Erythema toxicum

Fig. 186 Although the head and neck are the sites most commonly involved, port wine stains may occur anywhere. The lesions which are present from birth are permanent and histologically consist of dilated capillary vessels confined to the dermis.

Fig. 187 Erythema toxicum is a common neonatal eruption consisting of erythematous macules and small pustules containing eosinophils. The lesions fade and reappear at other sites but are quite benign. They should be distinguished from the more serious pustules of staphylococcal disease.

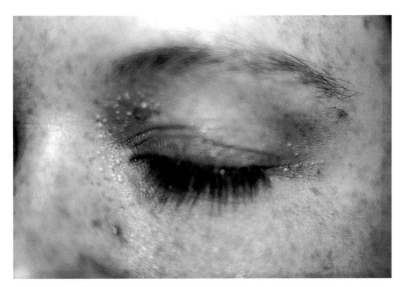

Fig. 188 Milia

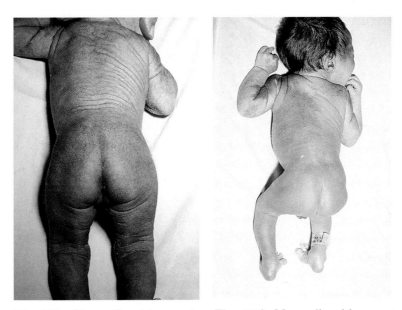

Fig. 189a Mongolian blue spot   **Fig. 189b Mongolian blue spot**

Fig. 188 Milia are small superficial keratin cysts which are common in neonates but which occur at all ages. The lesions are white, about 1–2 mm in diameter, and are often found on the cheeks and eyelids.

Fig. 189a–b Mongolian blue spot is common in children of African and Asian origin but can occur in Caucasians. The commonest sites are the lumbosacral areas and buttocks, but any area of skin may be affected. Lesions may be very extensive but gradually fade. It is important to distinguish blue spot from bruising, to avoid an incorrect diagnosis of non-accidental injury.

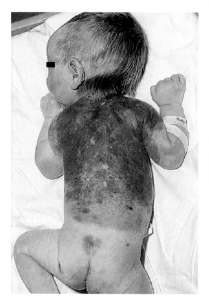

Fig. 190 Giant pigmented naevi

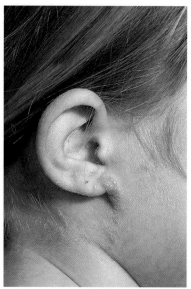

Fig. 191 Epidermal naevus

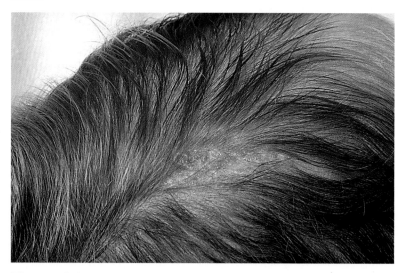

Fig. 192 Sebaceous naevus

Fig. 190 Giant pigmented naevi are extensive lesions which present at birth as deeply pigmented hairy areas, usually on the back or buttocks. As well as being disfiguring, there is a significant risk of malignant melanoma developing. Therefore, surgical excision, where possible, is indicated.

Fig. 191 This girl has a solitary, brownish, warty, linear naevus affecting the earlobe and adjacent skin. These lesions may present at birth or appear in the first month of life. Treatment, when required, is by surgical excision.

Fig. 192 A small, oval-shaped, slightly raised, yellow/orange hairless plaque is seen on the scalp. Sebaceous naevi, which contain sebaceous glands and all elements of skin, occur mainly on the head and neck of young children. Malignant change is common in adulthood and the lesions should be excised in adolescence.

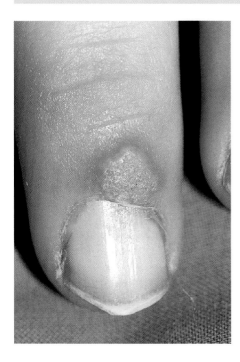

Fig. 193 Warts

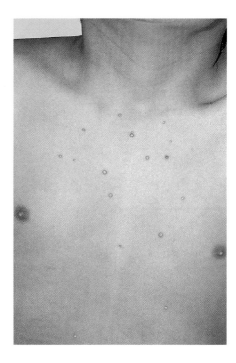

Fig. 194 Molluscum contagiosum

Fig. 193 Warts are caused by human papilloma viruses and are very common in children. Periungal lesions consisting of well-demarcated papules with a rough irregular surface are particularly common and show a predilection to occur at traumatised sites. Warts also occur on the face, knees and elbows. Most lesions disappear spontaneously within 3 years.

Fig. 194 Molluscum contagiosum is characterised by a number of small, discrete, dome-shaped, skin-coloured papules, which in this case are seen on the chest wall. These lesions are usually multiple and can appear anywhere, but the face, neck, axilla, trunk and anogenital region are common sites. These benign lesions are due to a pox virus and disappear spontaneously. Children with eczema are more prone to develop these lesions.

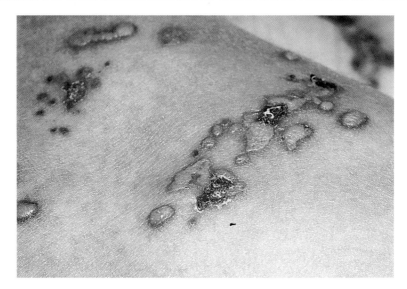

Fig. 195a Neonatal herpes simplex infection

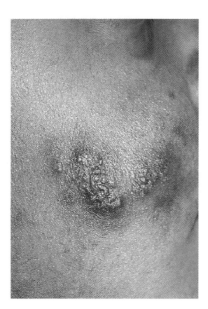

Fig. 195b Herpes simplex infection

Fig. 195a–b (**a**) In neonatal herpes simplex infection, vesicular skin lesions accompanied by erythema can occur at any site. They may ulcerate rapidly and often recur. Although skin lesions may be the only feature, disseminated disease with visceral involvement can occur with a high mortality. The infection is acquired from a mother with genital herpes during vaginal delivery. (**b**) In addition to the 'cold sore', recurrent herpes simplex virus infections can occur on the face, usually consisting of a crop of vesicles on an erythematous base. Exposure to sunlight and fever are precipitating factors. Herpes simplex infection is distinguished from herpes zoster by the absence of a dermatomal distribution.

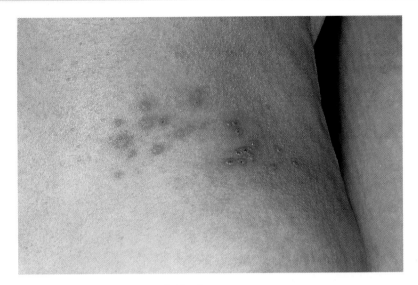

Fig. 196a Herpes zoster infection

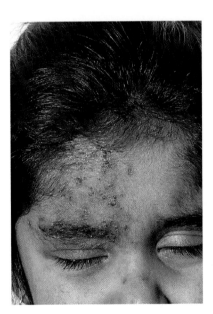

Fig. 196b Herpes zoster infection

Fig. 196a–b (**a**) A unilateral cluster of vesicular lesions with crusting is seen here in a dermatomal distribution. The rash is usually accompanied by localised pain, hyperaesthesia and pruritus. Herpes zoster infection is usually mild in normal children, but much more extensive disease occurs in immunocompromised patients, and intravenous acyclovir is necessary in this situation. (**b**) Vesicles on an erythematous background are present in the dermatomal distribution of the first division of the trigeminal nerve. Groups of vesicles may continue to appear for several weeks, but postherpetic neuralgia is very uncommon in children.

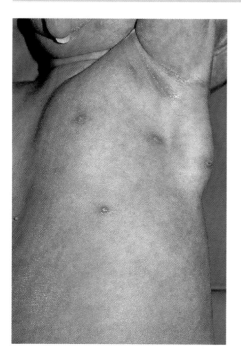

Fig. 197 Chickenpox

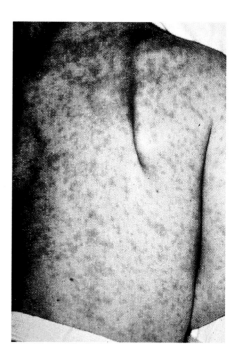

Fig. 198 Measles

Fig. 197 Often, the first sign of chickenpox is the appearance of vesicles on the trunk, scalp or face. Systemic upset is minimal. New lesions erupt for 4 or 5 days; the vesicles then become crusted. Occasionally, lesions occur in the mouth. This very common infection is much more serious in the immunocompromised child.

Fig. 198 In this case of measles, an extensive maculopapular rash is present over the back which is characteristically confluent at the back of the neck. The rash usually begins on the lateral aspects of the neck, along the hairline and behind the ears, and quickly spreads over the face, upper arms and upper chest during the following 24 hours. During the next 24 hours, the rash spreads to involve the back, abdomen and legs. After about 3 days the rash begins to fade, leaving a brown discoloration which lasts for several days.

Fig. 199 Erythema infectiosum

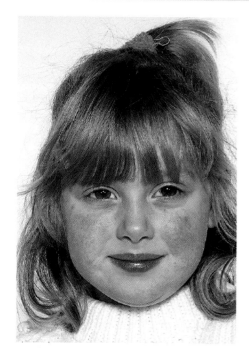

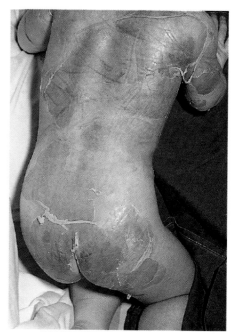

Fig. 200 Staphylococcal scalded skin syndrome

Fig. 199 Erythema infectiosum, also known as Fifth disease, is due to human parvovirus. Fever and pharyngitis are followed by a characteristic rash which gives a 'slapped cheek' appearance on the face. An erythematous rash is also seen on the extremities and trunk.

Fig. 200 Extensive denuded areas of skin resembling scalds are seen in staphylococcal scalded skin syndrome, which affects predominantly infants and young children. Extensive peeling of the epidermis is preceded by erythema and flaccid bullae. The rash is caused by toxin produced by phage group 2 staphylococci. Treatment is with a Beta lactamase resistant penicillin and recovery is usually complete.

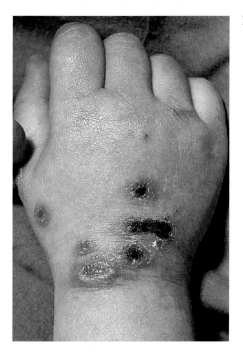

Fig. 201a Impetigo

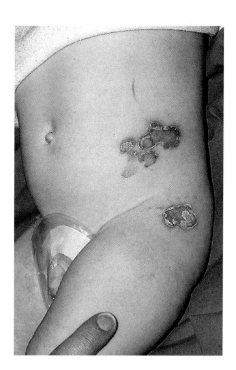

Fig. 201b Impetigo

Fig. 201a–b These skin lesions are usually caused by *Staphylococcus aureus*, and less often by β-haemolytic *Streptococcus*. Initial blisters quickly rupture to form crusted circular lesions with a moist eroded centre. The face and limbs are the most commonly affected sites. Occasionally, smaller crater-like lesions can be mistaken for cigarette burns.

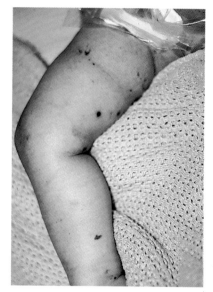

Fig. 202a Meningococcal septicaemia

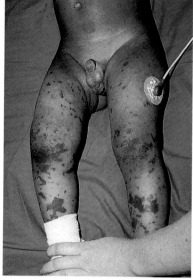

Fig. 202b Meningococcal septicaemia

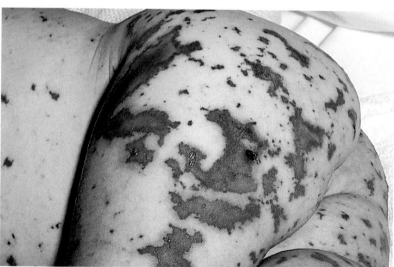

Fig. 202c Meningococcal septicaemia

Fig. 202a–c (**a**) A number of purpuric lesions are present on the limbs of this child who presented with fever and lethargy. This rash may be associated with meningitis. However, in the absence of meningeal involvement, meningococcal septicaemia often runs a more fulminant course with a worse prognosis. The rash may be very subtle at presentation and a careful search is indicated in any ill febrile child. (**b**) Widespread petechial and purpuric lesions are seen in this child with meningococcaemia and meningitis. The rash is sometimes atypical and erythematous. Antibiotics should be given immediately, and referral to an intensive care unit is often necessary. (**c**) In severe cases, extensive skin necrosis may develop. Shock is common and deterioration can be very rapid in meningococcaemia. Blood culture may be positive in 50% of cases, but the organism may be cultured from skin lesions and nasopharynx. Lumbar puncture may be hazardous to a patient in shock.

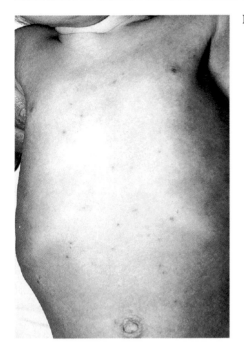

Fig. 203 Typhoid

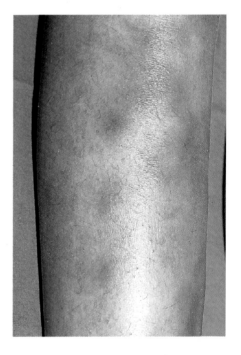

Fig. 204 Erythema nodosum

Fig. 203 In this case of typhoid, a characteristic discrete macular erythematous rash (rose spots) is seen. This rash usually appears during the second week of the illness and takes the form of crops of small skin lesions on the lower chest and abdomen. The rash usually lasts 2 or 3 days. *Salmonella* may be cultured from the lesions.

Fig. 204 These painful, red, hot, shiny nodules occur most frequently on the shins, although uncommonly they may occur on the buttocks, thighs and upper extremities. After a week or two, they fade to leave brown staining. The lesions occur in streptococcal infection, tuberculosis, inflammatory bowel disease, sarcoidosis and with drugs, particularly sulphonamides and oral contraceptives.

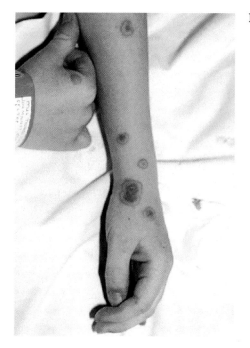

Fig. 205 Erythema multiforme

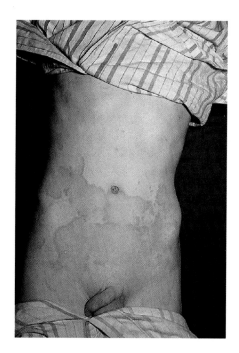

Fig. 206 Erythema marginatum

Fig. 205 Erythema multiforme is a hypersensitivity reaction associated with infections, particularly herpes simplex and *Mycoplasma* infection and drugs. Characteristic target lesions occur mainly on the extremities. In the more severe form, the Stevens–Johnson syndrome, the skin lesions are bullous, mucosal lesions occur at more than one site and systemic toxicity is present.

Fig. 206 Erythematous rings with pale centres are present on the trunk of this child. Erythema marginatum is probably specific for rheumatic fever but occurs in only 10–20% of cases. The rings which coalesce to form a changing pattern are found predominantly on the trunk and proximal parts of limbs.

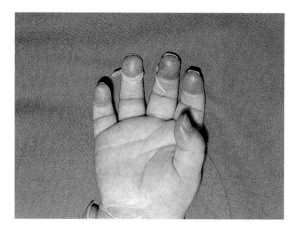

Fig. 207a Kawasaki syndrome

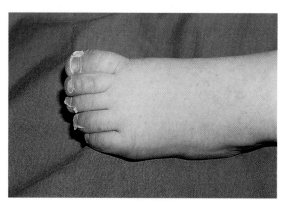

Fig. 207b Kawasaki syndrome

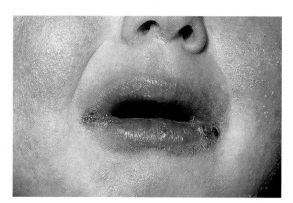

Fig. 207c Kawasaki syndrome

Fig. 207a–c The characteristic features of Kawasaki syndrome (mucocutaneous lymph node syndrome) are fever lasting more than 5 days, conjunctivitis, a generalised, usually erythematous, rash, involvement of mucous membranes of the upper respiratory tract, cervical lymphadenopathy and changes in the extremities including oedema and erythema. The diagnosis is made if fever of more than 5 days duration and four of the other features are present. Other illnesses such as staphylococcal and streptococcal disease should be excluded. The illustrations show desquamation of the hands and feet (**a,b**), which begins 10–20 days after the onset, and red fissured lips (**c**), evidence of mucosal involvement. The most serious sequel of the syndrome is cardiovascular involvement, which occurs in 20–30% of cases. Coronary artery aneurysms may develop following acute coronary arteritis.

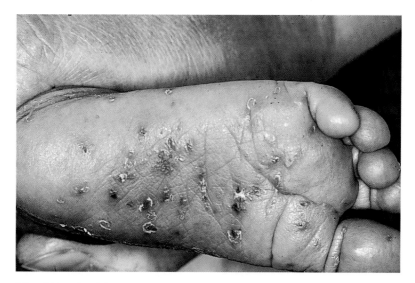

Fig. 208a Scabies

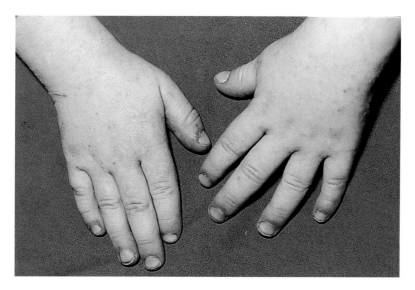

Fig. 208b Scabies

Fig. 208a–b (**a**) An intensely pruritic eruption is present on the sole, consisting of multiple papules and nodules with excoriation, scaling and crusting. This is due to infestation with *Sarcoptes scabiei*. In contrast to older children, scabies in infants often involves the soles, heels, arms, head and neck. The rash can be more widespread and burrows are more difficult to find. In older children, the eruption tends to affect the finger webs, flexor surface of the wrists, axillary folds and genitalia. (**b**) Several itchy papules are seen on the dorsum of the left hand and there is a burrow on the dorsum of the right hand. Scabies may be complicated by secondary infection (staphylococcal or streptococcal) and eczematous dermatitis.

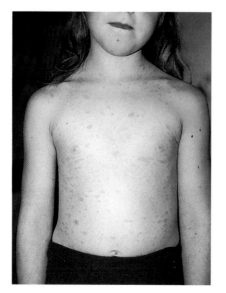

Fig. 209 Pityriasis rosea

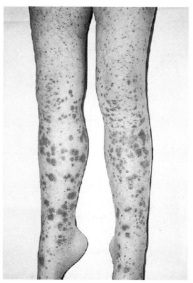

Fig. 210a Henoch–Schönlein purpura

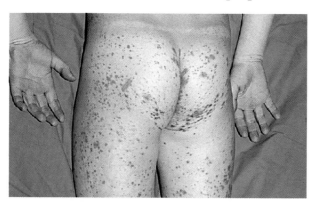

Fig. 210b Henoch–Schönlein purpura

Fig. 209 This girl with pityriasis rosea has a number of round or oval red papules on her trunk. The lesions characteristically become slightly scaly. The trunk is mainly involved and the oval patches often occur with their long axes running parallel to the ribs ('Christmas tree' distribution). The main rash is often preceded by a herald patch which occurs about 1 week earlier. This benign condition, which is thought to be viral in aetiology, resolves within a few weeks.

Fig. 210a–b A characteristic purpuric rash is present on this patient's legs and buttocks. The rash virtually always involves the lower limbs, and often the buttocks and extensor surfaces of the arms, but may be absent at the latter two sites. It begins as a red maculopapular rash and then becomes purpuric. The skin lesions are variable and may be urticarial. Itching is not a feature. The purpuric lesions eventually become brown before fading. They often appear in crops. Angioedema may also be present, especially in younger children. The other features of Henoch–Schönlein purpura are involvement of the gastrointestinal tract (abdominal pain, vomiting, haematemesis, melaena), glomerulonephritis and arthritis.

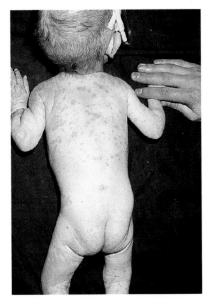

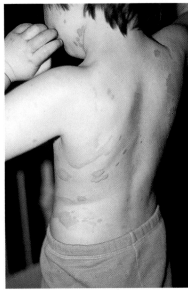

Fig. 211 Cow's milk protein intolerance

Fig. 212a Urticaria

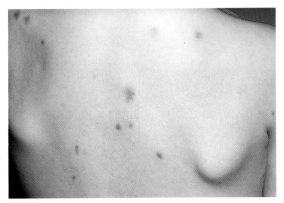

Fig. 212b Urticaria pigmentosa

Fig. 211 Wasting and a generalised rash can be seen in this boy who presented with vomiting, diarrhoea and failure to thrive. His symptoms resolved with the exclusion of cow's milk. In some cases of cow's milk protein intolerance, a patchy enteropathy is found on small intestinal biopsy. In others, occult faecal blood loss may lead to anaemia.

Fig. 212a–b (a) This girl has a number of itchy erythematous raised skin lesions of varying size (wheals). Urticaria is a common condition which may be caused by foods, drugs, inhalants, infectious agents or physical factors, but often a cause cannot be identified. Allergy testing is usually unhelpful. Urticaria is usually a benign self-limiting condition for which antihistamines are the only treatment necessary. (b) In urticaria pigmentosa, small red brown papules or macules occur, usually on the trunk, in the first year of life. The lesions urticate easily when rubbed due to the presence of large numbers of mast cells. Treatment is not required as the lesions resolve spontaneously.

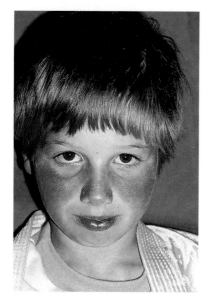

Fig. 213a Systemic lupus erythematosus

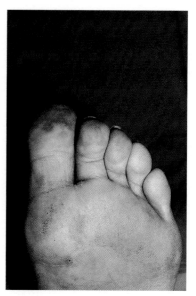

Fig. 213b Systemic lupus erythematosus

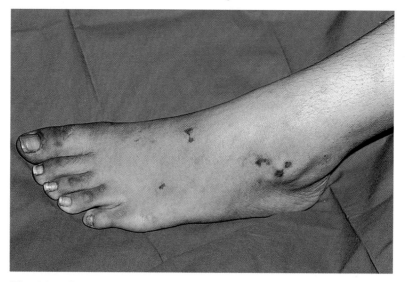

Fig. 213c Systemic lupus erythematosus

Fig. 213a–c (**a**) This girl shows the characteristic malar or butterfly erythematous rash of systemic lupus erythematosus (SLE). The rash usually spares the nasolabial folds and is photosensitive. Arthralgia or arthritis and rash are the commonest presenting features in children. (**b,c**) Peripheral blood vessel involvement can be severe in SLE. This girl presented with vasculitic skin lesions of both feet and a history of fatigue and arthralgia for several months. The lesions resolved with large doses of corticosteroids.

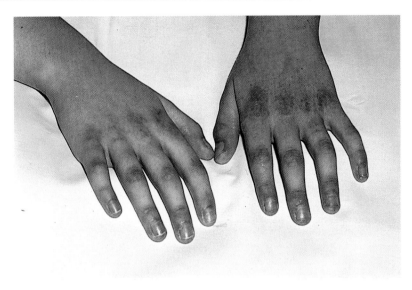

Fig. 214a Dermatomyositis

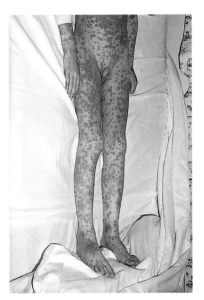

Fig. 214b Dermatomyositis

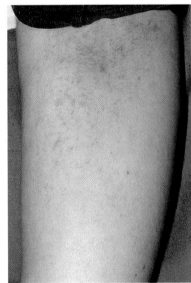

**Fig. 215 Systemic onset
juvenile chronic arthritis**

Fig. 214a–b (**a**) In this case of dermatomyositis, erythematous patches are present over the extensor surfaces of the fingers. Erythematous skin lesions occur elsewhere but mainly on the upper eyelids, malar region, elbows and knees. Muscle weakness is usually proximal and symmetrical. Myalgia and proximal muscle tenderness may also be present. (**b**) This patient also has extensive erythematous lesions on his limbs and trunk.

Fig. 215 Most children with systemic onset juvenile chronic arthritis (Still's disease) have an intermittent rash which usually consists of small pink macules occurring mainly on the trunk and limbs. The rash, which often comes and goes with fever, and other systemic features such as anaemia, hepatosplenomegaly and lymphadenopathy often precede the development of arthritis.

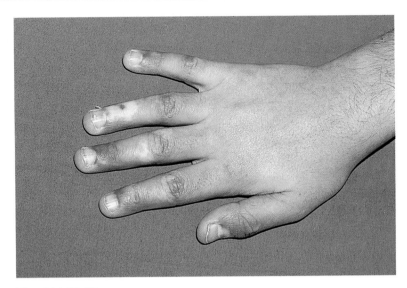

Fig. 216 Vitiligo

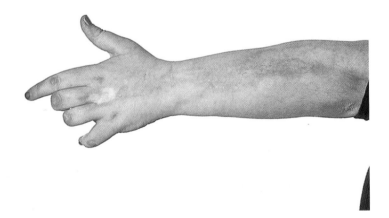

Fig. 217 Linear scleroderma

Fig. 216 Vitiligo is a common disorder which consists of multiple, sharply demarcated areas of depigmented skin. The lesions are often symmetrical but can be unilateral. Common sites are hands, feet, around the mouth or eyes, neck and axillae, but almost anywhere can be affected. A positive family history is common and there is an association with autoimmune disorders.

Fig. 217 A band of sclerosis is seen affecting the length of the arm and associated with contractures of the fingers. Although localised, linear scleroderma can be quite disfiguring, with involvement of underlying musculoskeletal structures and impairment of function. Hemiatrophy is a common sequel.

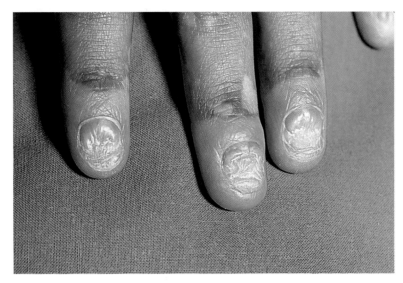

Fig. 218a Chronic mucocutaneous candidiasis

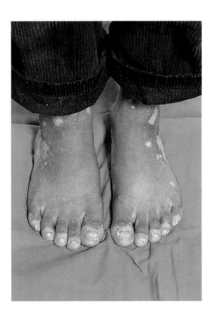

Fig. 218b Chronic mucocutaneous candidiasis

Fig. 218a–b Chronic mucocutaneous candidiasis, due to a selective immune defect in handling *Candida*, affects the oral cavity, nails, hands and feet. Misshapen hypertrophic nails can be seen in addition to vitiligo. Other autoimmune disorders such as hypoparathyroidism, Addison's disease and hypothyroidism may occur.

Fig. 219a Tuberous sclerosis

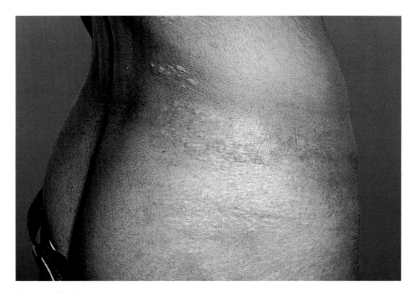

Fig. 219b Tuberous sclerosis

Fig. 219a–c (**a**) A depigmented macule is present on the trunk of this baby who presented with seizures. Often described as like a 'mountain ash leaf', these lesions often occur in the first year and are best visualised with ultraviolet (Wood's) light. They are not specific for tuberous sclerosis (TS) and may occur in normal children. (**b**) Shagreen patches, which are highly characteristic of TS, are large, thickened, discoloured, leathery, plaque-like lesions. They occur in the lumbosacral region, usually to one side of the midline, and are present in 40% of TS patients. (**c**, opposite) This child has facial angiofibromas (formerly referred to as adenoma sebaceum) which consist of red/pink nodules distributed symmetrically and bilaterally over the cheeks in a butterfly distribution and on the chin. The upper lip is usually spared. These lesions affect 85% of patients with TS but are rarely seen before the age of 3 years. They usually become more prominent at puberty.

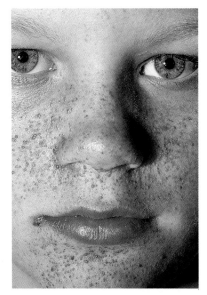

Fig. 219c Tuberous sclerosis

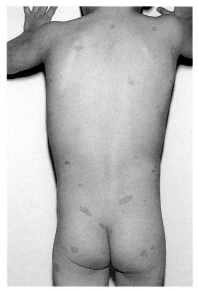

Fig. 220a Neurofibromatosis
type I

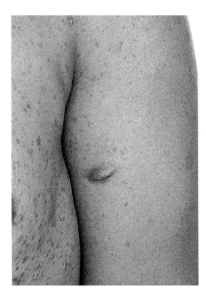

Fig. 220b Neurofibromatosis
type I

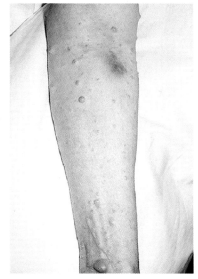

Fig. 220c Neurofibromatosis
type I

Fig. 220a–c (**a**) This patient with neurofibromatosis type I has several café-au-lait patches on his trunk. To make this diagnosis, there should be more than six café-au-lait spots over 5 mm in diameter in the pre-pubertal child (or over 15 mm in the postpubertal patient) plus two or more of the following: axillary freckling, peripheral neurofibromata, plexiform neurofibroma, typical bony lesions, Lisch nodules or an affected family member. (**b**) Typical axillary freckling can be seen in this patient who had many café-au-lait patches. A neurofibroma is seen on the upper part of the left arm. (**c**) Multiple dermal neurofibromas, consisting of nodules of varying sizes, are present along the paths of peripheral nerves on this patient's arm. Dermal neurofibromas usually make their appearance at puberty and gradually become more numerous with increasing age.

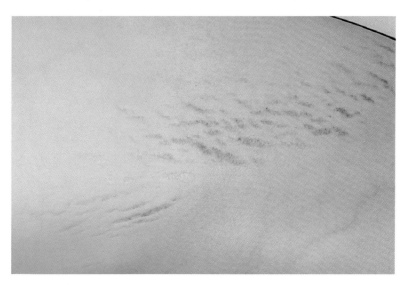

Fig. 221 Striae

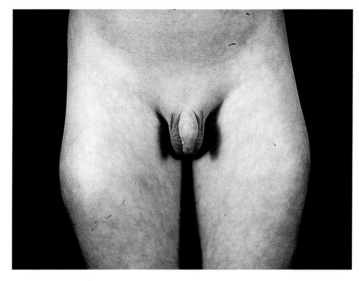

Fig. 222 Lipohypertrophy

Fig. 221 Purple red bands of thin atrophic skin are seen. These will eventually become paler, smoother and silvery. They occur at sites of skin stretching, particularly the abdomen, lower back, breasts, thighs and around the axillae. Rapid growth, obesity and pregnancy are the commonest causes. Less commonly, striae are caused by Cushing's syndrome and prolonged corticosteroid treatment. Although permanent, they may become less conspicuous with time.

Fig. 222 Areas of fat hypertrophy are seen on the lateral aspects of the thighs in this diabetic boy. These occur at overused injection sites and can adversely affect diabetic control because insulin absorption is irregular. Like lipoatrophy, this has also become less common with the use of purer insulins and rotation of the injection site.

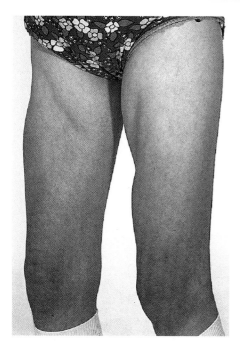

Fig. 223 Diabetic lipoatrophy

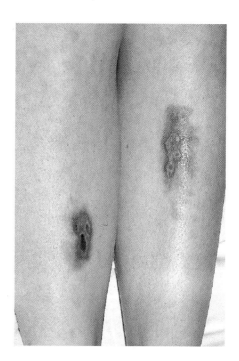

Fig. 224 Necrobiosis lipoidica

Fig. 223 Skin depressions are seen on both thighs of this diabetic girl due to loss of fat. Frequent rotation of the sites of insulin injection reduces the incidence of this complication which has become less common since the introduction of human insulins.

Fig. 224 Necrobiosis lipoidica is a disorder of the dermal connective tissue and occurs almost exclusively in diabetes. The lesions are usually found on the pretibial areas and consist of erythematous plaques with atrophic centres. The lesions develop into sclerotic plaques. Ulceration may occur.

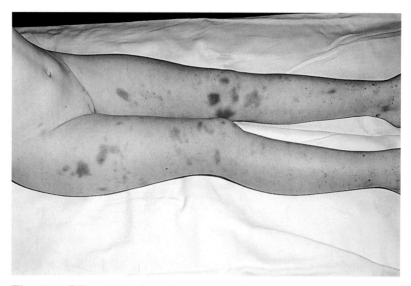

Fig. 225a Idiopathic thrombocytopaenic purpura

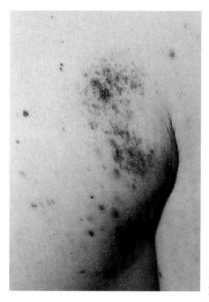

Fig. 225b Idiopathic thrombocytopaenic purpura

Fig. 225a–b The clinical features of idiopathic thrombocytopaenic purpura are usually confined to superficial bruising and a petechial rash. The petechiae do not blanch on pressure. Bleeding from mucous membranes may occur, but more serious bleeding such as intracranial haemorrhage is very rare. Hepatosplenomegaly and lymphadenopathy are not features and should point to other diagnoses, particularly acute leukaemia. The platelet count is usually $<20 \times 10^9$/L in the presence of widespread bruising and petechiae. The prognosis is excellent even if no treatment is given. If treatment with steroids is contemplated, a bone marrow examination should be performed to exclude leukaemia. Corticosteroids alone given to a patient with acute leukaemia temporarily mask the disease and jeopardise survival.

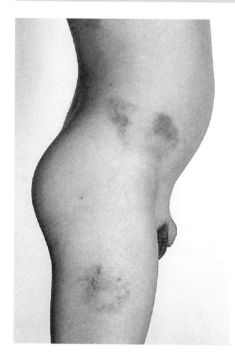

Fig. 226 Haemophilia

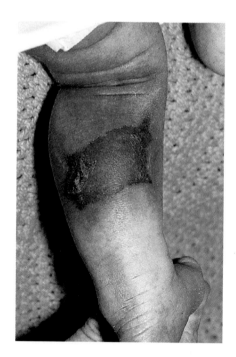

Fig. 227 Protein C deficiency

Fig. 226 Although haematoma and haemarthrosis are the hallmarks of haemophilia, an increased tendency to bruising often occurs, particularly in the active younger child. Such bruising is often more extensive and 'colourful' than in normal children.

Fig. 227 An area of skin necrosis is seen on the calf of this baby with homozygous protein C deficiency. In addition to skin lesions (purpura fulminans), these infants often have eye complications due to retinal artery and vein thrombosis and neurological complications which may lead to death or handicap.

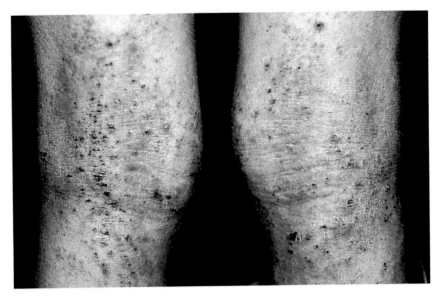

Fig. 228a Eczema

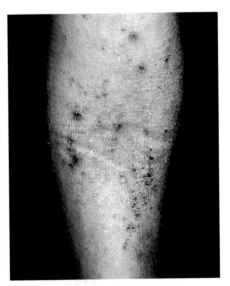

Fig. 228b Eczema

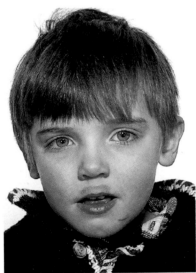

Fig. 228c Lick eczema

Fig. 228a–e (**a,b**) Excoriated erythematous papular lesions are present behind the knee and in the antecubital fossa. These lesions are intensely pruritic, and scratching leads to weeping and crusting. Secondary infection is common. Eczema often begins in infancy, with involvement of the face, neck, hands, abdomen and extensor surfaces. Characteristically, involvement of flexor surfaces appears later. Continued involvement of the extensor surfaces often indicates more troublesome eczema. (**c**) Lick eczema is a contact irritant dermatitis due to the habit of lip licking. The rash resolves when the child abandons the habit. (**d,e**, opposite) Eczema herpeticum is the result of herpes simplex infection in children with atopic eczema. Infection, which may be widespread, begins with groups of vesicles, but crusting and erosions often follow. Fever and systemic upset may occur. Treatment with acyclovir is necessary.

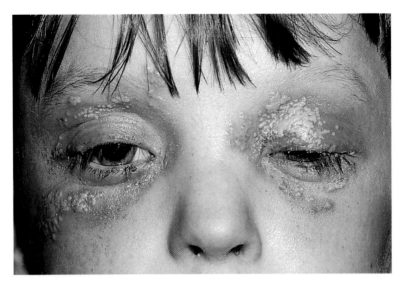

Fig. 228d Eczema herpeticum

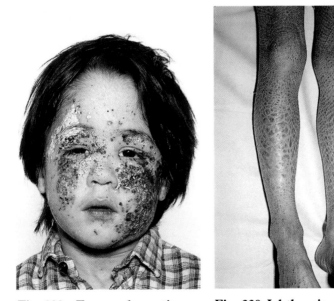

Fig. 228e Eczema herpeticum   **Fig. 229 Ichthyosis vulgaris**

Fig. 229 Large scales can be seen over the shins of this patient. Ichthyosis vulgaris is the common-est of the different forms of ichthyosis. Scaling often affects the extensor surfaces of the extremities, with sparing of the flexors. Atopic eczema is a common accompanying disorder.

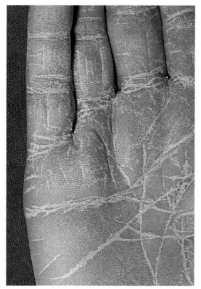

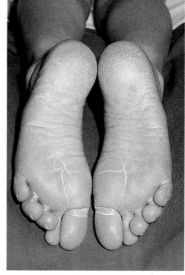

Fig. 230a Hyperkeratosis   **Fig. 230b Hyperkeratosis**

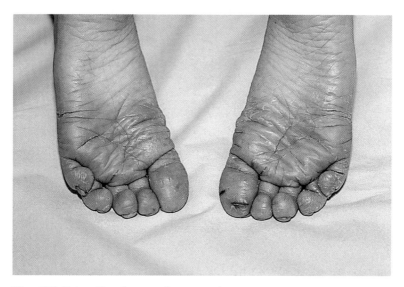

Fig. 231 Juvenile plantar dermatosis

Fig. 230a–b Dry, thickened and wrinkled skin is present in this child with hyperkeratosis of the palms and soles. This is seen in several of the different types of ichthyosis.

Fig. 231 Juvenile plantar dermatosis is a recently recognised dermatitis caused by synthetic footwear with poor moisture absorption. The toes and forefoot are affected and occasionally the heel. The affected skin is dry, cracked, glazed and painful. Peeling often occurs.

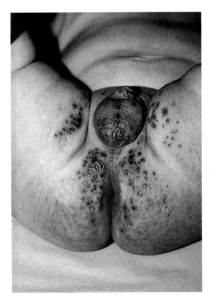

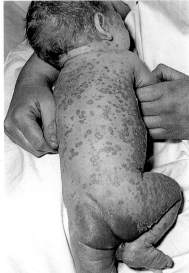

Fig. 232 Napkin dermatitis   **Fig. 233 Psoriasis**

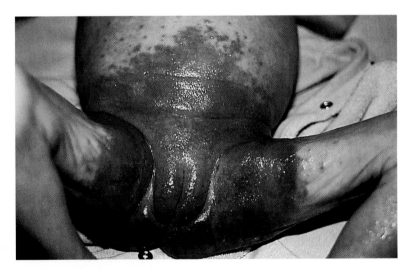

Fig. 234 Napkin rash due to candidiasis

Fig. 232 Redness and superficial erosions are present in the napkin area. This is an irritant contact dermatitis due to contact with urine, faeces or irritant chemicals in inadequately rinsed nappies. The skin folds are characteristically spared.

Fig. 233 This infant has a generalised rash consisting of slightly raised erythematous scaly plaques with more extensive involvement of the napkin area. Typical psoriasis is uncommon in the first 2 years of life. The disease often starts in the napkin area but extends outwards. The lesions may resolve spontaneously, although recurrence can occur later in childhood.

Fig. 234 In this napkin rash due to candidiasis, there is an unusually florid erythematous monilial rash with satellite lesions and lack of sparing of skin folds. Muscle wasting and abdominal distension are also seen in this child who was severely immunosuppressed and had persistent chronic diarrhoea.

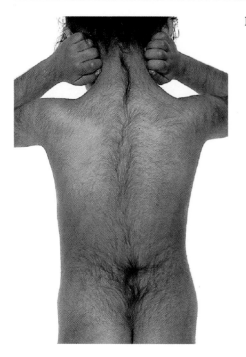

Fig. 235 Hirsutism

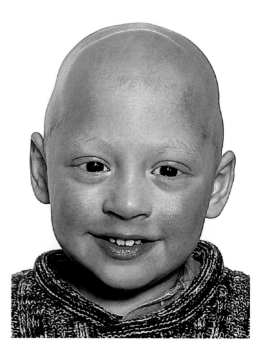

Fig. 236 Alopecia areata

Fig. 235 Excessive hair growth is seen on this girl's back due to cyclosporin. Other causes of generalised hirsutism include other drugs, e.g. phenytoin and corticosteroids, endocrine disorders such as virilising ovarian and adrenal tumours, and a number of congenital syndromes. Mild hirsutism is commonly racial or familial.

Fig. 236 This boy has total hair loss from his scalp (alopecia totalis). This condition is sometimes familial but often no cause is apparent. Alopecia areata may be associated in some cases with atopy or autoimmune disease. Prognosis is good with few patches of hair loss but must be guarded if hair loss is extensive.

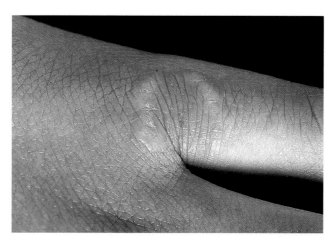

Fig. 237 Granuloma annulare

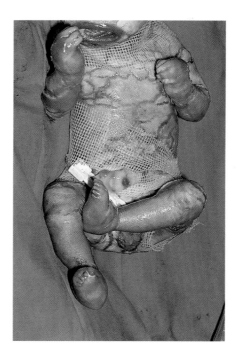

Fig. 238 Harlequin fetus

Fig. 237 There is a ring-like papule overlying the 5th metacarpophalangeal joint. The lesions of granuloma annulare are asymptomatic and may occur at any site but are commonly found over bony prominences, especially over the back of the hands and feet. The lesions begin as red smooth papules and then enlarge to form annular plaques which often have a beaded appearance. The aetiology is unknown and lesions usually disappear spontaneously.

Fig. 238 In cases of harlequin fetus, a rare autosomal recessive disorder, markedly thickened cracked skin forms disfiguring plaques over the entire body. Facial features are grotesque, with everted gapping lips and severe ectropion. Limb movement and respiratory movement are restricted. Most babies are stillborn or die soon after birth.

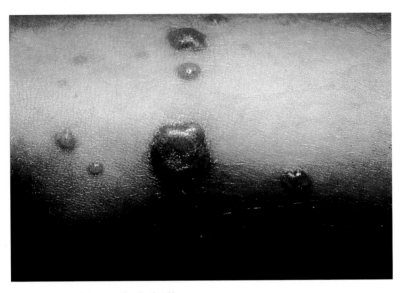

Fig. 239 Epidermolysis bullosa

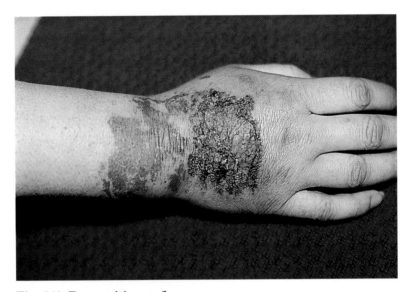

Fig. 240 Dermatitis artefacta

Fig. 239 Several haemorrhagic blisters are seen in this case of epidermolysis bullosa. The characteristic feature of this group of disorders is the appearance of blisters with mechanical, often mild, trauma or warm weather. The autosomal dominant types such as epidermolysis bullosa simplex are generally milder than the more severe recessively inherited types.

Fig. 240 Unusual skin lesions which are bizarre and do not conform to any recognised skin conditions may be self-inflicted. The site is always one which is easily accessible to self-inflicted injury. Dermatitis artefacta, which is commoner in older girls, may represent a form of attention-seeking.

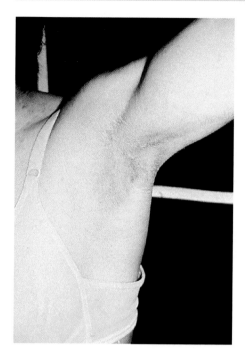

Fig. 241 Acanthosis nigricans

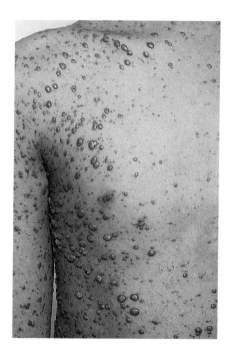

Fig. 242 Xanthoma disseminatum

Fig. 241 A hyperpigmented, hyperkeratotic plaque is seen in the axilla of this patient. These plaques are most often found in the axilla, groin and neck, but can occur virtually anywhere. Acanthosis nigricans is associated with obesity, diabetes and other endocrine disorders. It may occasionally be familial.

Fig. 242 This boy has a large number of xanthomata consisting of brown nodules involving most of his trunk, arms, neck and face. The skin lesions in this rare condition may regress spontaneously after months or years. Diabetes insipidus due to pituitary involvement and mucous membrane involvement is common. This boy has extensive involvement with panhypopituitarism, laryngeal involvement causing hoarseness and intracranial lesions.

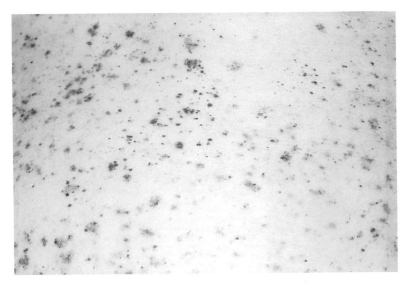

Fig. 243 Letterer–Siwe disease

Fig. 243 The typical rash in Letterer–Siwe disease consists of purpuric lesions amidst a seborrhoeic dermatitis-like background. A widespread rash may be present before the onset of other features such as fever, hepatosplenomegaly and lymphadenopathy. Letterer–Siwe disease, eosinophilic granuloma and Hand–Schüller–Christian disease are now referred to as Langerhans cell histiocytosis.

6 Child abuse

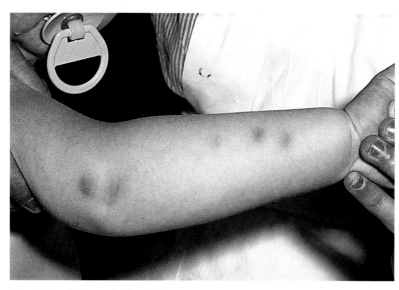

Fig. 244a Fingertip bruising

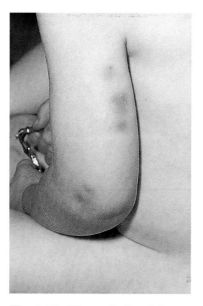

Fig. 244b Fingertip bruising

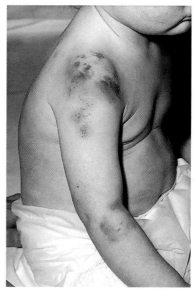

Fig. 245 Bruises of different ages

Fig. 244a–b Multiple round bruises are seen on this baby's lower arm (**a**). They have been caused by forceful gripping between thumb and fingers of one hand. Usually, bruising from the fingertips is more prominent than bruising from the thumb. The presence of fingertip bruising on the posterior aspects of both upper arms or around the chest wall often suggests that the child has been shaken (**b**). A search must then be made for retinal haemorrhages and/or evidence of intracranial bleeding.

Fig. 245 Multiple bruises of varying age are seen on this child's upper arm. Multiple bruising is often inconsistent with the history provided and bruising of different colours indicates more than one episode.

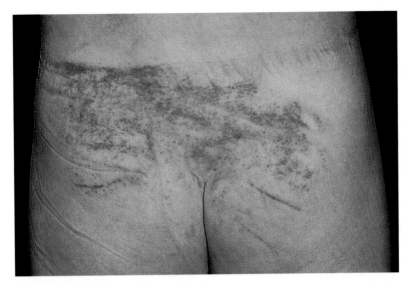

Fig. 246 Bruising on the buttocks

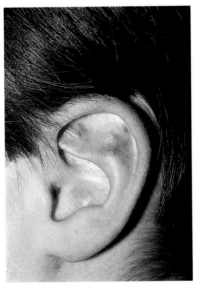

Fig. 247a Ear bruising

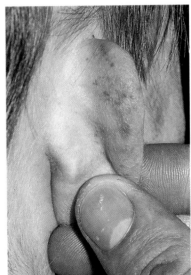

Fig. 247b Ear bruising

Fig. 246 Accidental bruising is less likely to occur on the buttocks, back and soft tissue areas such as the cheek. This child has extensive bruising of the buttocks, and linear bruises can be seen indicating that he has been beaten.

Fig. 247a–b Bruising involving the anterior and posterior surfaces of the helix of the ear is a common finding in physically abused children. These are not sites where accidental bruising usually occurs. The bruises are usually caused by cuffing.

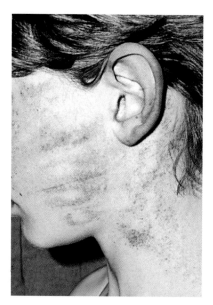

Fig. 248 Slap marks

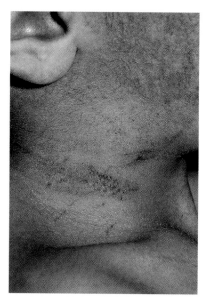

Fig. 249a Strangulation

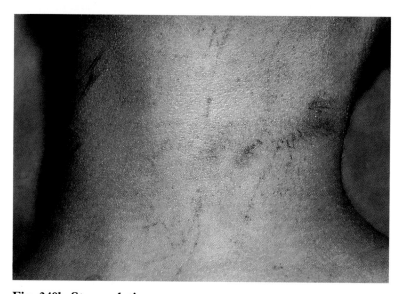

Fig. 249b Strangulation

Fig. 248 There are a number of linear red marks on the left side of the face and neck due to slapping. The red lines represent capillary outlining or the 'tramlining' effect in which blood from damaged capillaries is displaced outwards from the point of impact. As most people are right-handed, most slap marks occur on the left side of the face.

Fig. 249a–b Linear petechial bruising is present on both sides and the front and back of this child's neck, caused by attempted strangulation. Petechial bruising can be seen on the lower part of his face. This in fact was extensive, covering most of his face and forehead, and was due to asphyxiation.

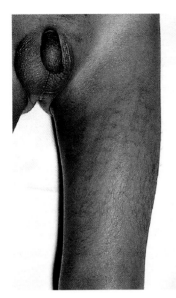

Fig. 250 Bruising caused by a trainer

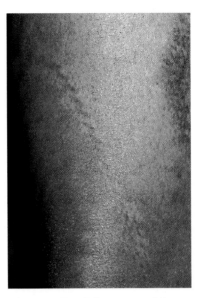

Fig. 251 Bruising caused by a dog leash

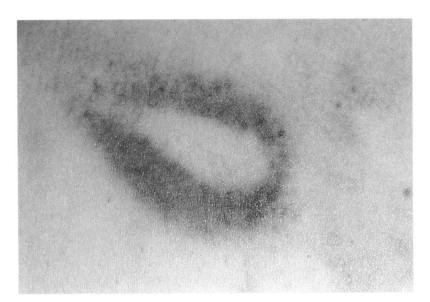

Fig. 252 Bruising caused by a wooden spoon

Fig. 250 A clear imprint of the sole of a trainer can be detected in the bruise on this boy's thigh.

Fig. 251 The braided pattern of a cord can be seen on this child's leg. The pattern was found to correspond to that on a dog lead found in the child's home.

Fig. 252 Bruising forming the clear outline of a wooden spoon is present. This child was struck with the convex surface of the spoon.

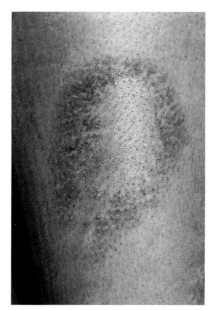

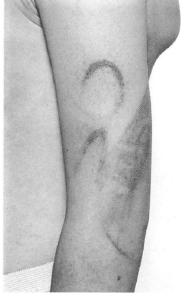

Fig. 253 Bruising caused by a carpet slipper

Fig. 254 Whip injury

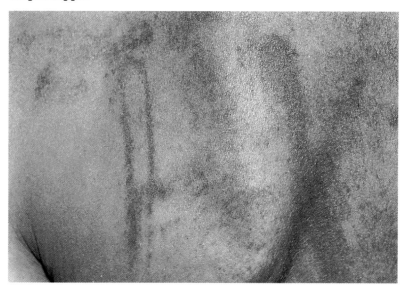

Fig. 255 Bruising caused by a cricket stump

Fig. 253 The imprint of the outer edge of the sole of a carpet slipper can be seen.

Fig. 254 Characteristic bruising caused by lashing with a looped cord or rope is seen on this child's arm. Lashing with a loop cord produces a clearly defined semicircular or oval-shaped bruise of uniform intensity.

Fig. 255 Multiple linear bruises are present where this boy has been hit with a cricket stump. Also seen is the 'tramlining' effect or capillary outlining. The point of impact is not bruised, but the adjoining skin on both sides shows bruising due to damaged capillaries.

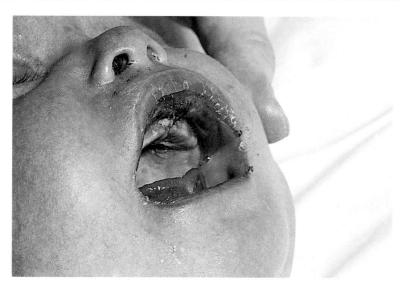

Fig. 256 Torn frenulum

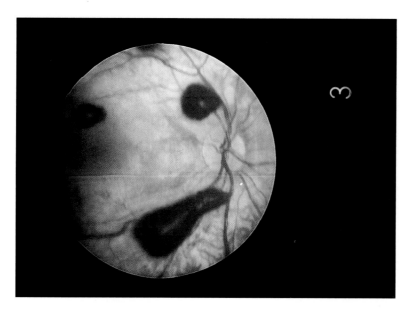

Fig. 257 Retinal haemorrhage

Fig. 256 A torn frenulum is very suggestive of child abuse. Often, an object such as a feeding cup is forced against this part of the mouth. However, some cases are the result of genuine accident, e.g. the toddler who falls against the edge of a small table.

Fig. 257 Extensive retinal haemorrhage is present due to acceleration/deceleration forces associated with shaking. Retinal haemorrhages may occur in neonates, but they disappear within a few days and their presence thereafter is a strong pointer towards abuse. There may be an associated brain injury; in particular, subdural haematoma should be excluded.

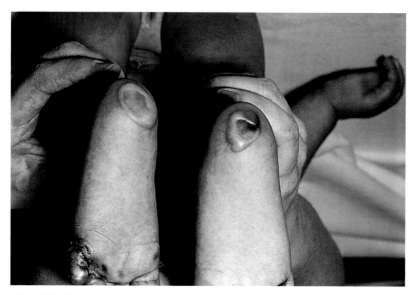

Fig. 258 Burns from a flat surface

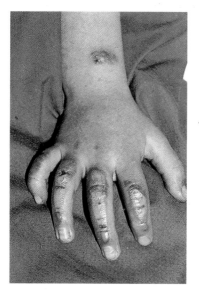

Fig. 259a Burns from a hot iron

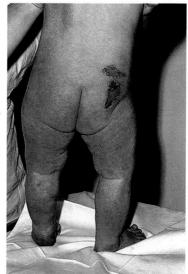

Fig. 259b Burn from a hot iron

Fig. 258 There are contact burns on the anterior and posterior parts on both soles. The child's feet were thought to have been placed on a hot cooking ring.

Fig. 259a–b (**a**) There are burns to the dorsal surfaces of the fingers, indicating contact with a hot flat surface, in this case a hot iron. Such burns on the dorsal surface are not likely to be accidental. Accidental burns to the hand are more likely to involve the palmar surface. (**b**) A triangular burn from contact with a hot iron is present on the buttocks. The child's parent was ironing clothes on the floor at the time when she inflicted the injury.

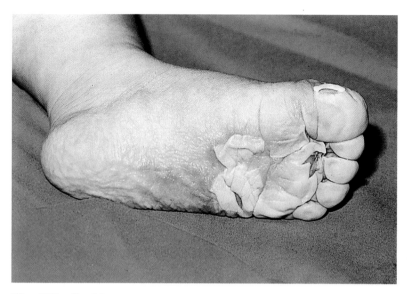

Fig. 260a Scalds

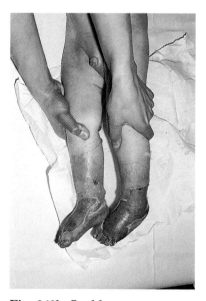

Fig. 260b Scalds

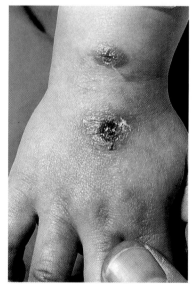

Fig. 261 Cigarette burns

Fig. 260a–b (**a**) There is full-thickness burning to the sole in this child whose foot was immersed in very hot water. (**b**) This child has immersion burns in a symmetrical stocking distribution which were sustained when she was lowered into a hot bath. Accidental scalds often involve the upper parts of the body, e.g. from pulling over a hot drink, and the scalds are often irregular with splash marks. The buttocks are also commonly involved in immersion burns.

Fig. 261 There is a deep punched-out crater on the dorsum of the hand, a typical site for non-accidental cigarette burns. This is not a particularly common form of abuse and may sometimes be difficult to distinguish from impetigo. Accidental cigarette burns usually consist of a circular mark and a tail and are less deep.

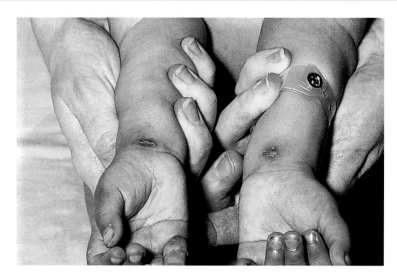

Fig. 262 Match burns

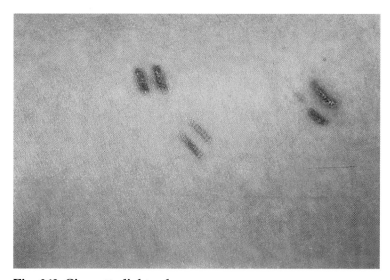

Fig. 263 Cigarette lighter burns

Fig. 262 Symmetrical burns are present on both wrists due to contact with a hot matchstick. These injuries, like many other non-accidental burns, represent serious abuse and suggest a sadistic intent on the part of the abuser. Symmetrical injuries may represent a ritualistic form of abuse.

Fig. 263 These three sets of parallel burns were inflicted on this child using the heated cogwheel of a disposable cigarette lighter. A ridged pattern was present in the brand marks corresponding to ridges on the lighter. This is also an example of serious sadistic abuse.

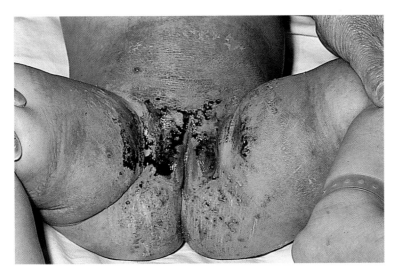

Fig. 264a Neglect

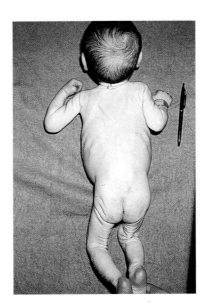

Fig. 264b Neglect

Fig. 264a–b (**a**) Severe nappy rash, often with ulcerated areas, may be a feature of neglect if a child is left for long periods in a wet and soiled nappy. The rash will often resolve rapidly during a hospital admission. (**b**) This baby is severely malnourished with very little subcutaneous tissue as a result of neglect. In such cases, head circumference and length may be appropriate for age unless neglect has been long-standing. The diagnosis is usually confirmed by hospital admission and demonstration of rapid weight gain.

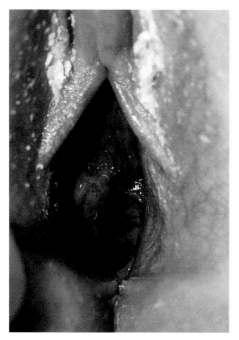

Fig. 265a Sexual abuse

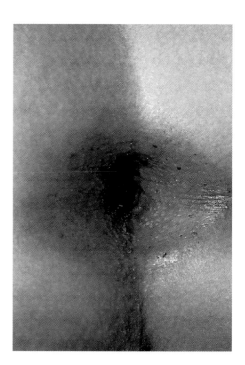

Fig. 265b Sexual abuse

Fig. 265a–b (**a**) A small tear is present at the posterior fourchette in this girl who disclosed sexual abuse. Abnormal physical findings are often absent or minimal in girls referred for examination for possible sexual abuse. In contrast to injuries caused by sexual abuse, accidental injuries to the vulva are more likely to occur anteriorly. (**b**) The anus is widely dilated on immediate parting of the buttocks in this boy who disclosed recent penile penetration by an older relative.

Index